Statistical Methods for Immunogenicity Assessment

Chapman & Hall/CRC Biostatistics Series

Published Titles

Adaptive Design Methods in Clinical Trials, Second Edition
Shein-Chung Chow and Mark Chang

Adaptive Designs for Sequential Treatment Allocation
Alessandro Baldi Antognini and Alessandra Giovagnoli

Adaptive Design Theory and Implementation Using SAS and R, Second Edition
Mark Chang

Advanced Bayesian Methods for Medical Test Accuracy
Lyle D. Broemeling

Advances in Clinical Trial Biostatistics
Nancy L. Geller

Applied Meta-Analysis with R
Ding-Geng (Din) Chen and Karl E. Peace

Basic Statistics and Pharmaceutical Statistical Applications, Second Edition
James E. De Muth

Bayesian Adaptive Methods for Clinical Trials
Scott M. Berry, Bradley P. Carlin, J. Jack Lee, and Peter Muller

Bayesian Analysis Made Simple: An Excel GUI for WinBUGS
Phil Woodward

Bayesian Methods for Measures of Agreement
Lyle D. Broemeling

Bayesian Methods in Epidemiology
Lyle D. Broemeling

Bayesian Methods in Health Economics
Gianluca Baio

Bayesian Missing Data Problems: EM, Data Augmentation and Noniterative Computation
Ming T. Tan, Guo-Liang Tian, and Kai Wang Ng

Bayesian Modeling in Bioinformatics
Dipak K. Dey, Samiran Ghosh, and Bani K. Mallick

Benefit-Risk Assessment in Pharmaceutical Research and Development
Andreas Sashegyi, James Felli, and Rebecca Noel

Biosimilars: Design and Analysis of Follow-on Biologics
Shein-Chung Chow

Biostatistics: A Computing Approach
Stewart J. Anderson

Causal Analysis in Biomedicine and Epidemiology: Based on Minimal Sufficient Causation
Mikel Aickin

Clinical and Statistical Considerations in Personalized Medicine
Claudio Carini, Sandeep Menon, and Mark Chang

Chapman & Hall/CRC Biostatistics Series

Statistical Methods for Immunogenicity Assessment

Harry Yang • Jianchun Zhang

Binbing Yu • Wei Zhao

MedImmune, LLC

Gaithersburg, Maryland, USA

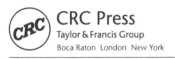

CRC Press

Taylor & Francis Group

Boca Raton London New York

CRC Press is an imprint of the
Taylor & Francis Group, an **informa** business

A CHAPMAN & HALL BOOK

CRC Press
Taylor & Francis Group
6000 Broken Sound Parkway NW, Suite 300
Boca Raton, FL 33487-2742

First issued in paperback 2020

ISBN-13: 978-1-4987-0034-4 (hbk)
ISBN-13: 978-0-367-73797-9 (pbk)

Library of Congress Cataloging-in-Publication Data

Yang, Harry, author.
    Statistical methods for immunogenicity assessment / Harry Yang, Jianchun Zhang, Binbing Yu, Wei Zhao.
        p. ; cm. -- (Chapman & Hall/CRC biostatistics series)
    Includes bibliographical references and index.
    ISBN 978-1-4987-0034-4 (hardcover : alk. paper)
    I. Zhang, Jianchun (Statistician), author. II. Yu, Binbing, author. III. Zhao, Wei, 1975- , author. IV. Title. V. Series: Chapman & Hall/CRC biostatistics series (Unnumbered)
    [DNLM: 1. Immunogenetic Phenomena. 2. Statistics as Topic. 3. Drug Design. 4. Risk Assessment--methods. QW 541]

QR186
615.7'040727--dc23   2015026245

Visit the Taylor & Francis Web site at
http://www.taylorandfrancis.com

and the CRC Press Web site at
http://www.crcpress.com

To our families

Contents

Preface

Biotechnology-derived therapeutics including monoclonal antibodies, proteins, and peptides hold great promise for treating various diseases such as cancer and inflammatory diseases. They also represent an important class of therapeutic interventions. However, because of their large size, complex structure, and complicated manufacture process, biopharmaceutical products can lead to immunogenic responses, resulting in formation of anti-drug antibodies (ADAs). Immune responses to non-vaccine biologics have the potential to negatively affect both patient safety and product efficacy. For example, a neutralizing antibody is deleterious if it inhibits the efficacy of the product, and can be harmful when it cross-reacts with an endogenous counterpart of the therapeutic in patients. Non-neutralizing antibodies may affect the pharmacokinetic properties of the drug, thus may affect dosing regime. These immunologically-based consequences may cause drug developers to either terminate development or limit the use of otherwise effective therapies. Therefore, immunogenicity assessment is a key component of biopharmaceutical safety and efficacy evaluation, and a prerequisite for the successful development of biopharmaceuticals. Furthermore, immunogenicity is also a complex phenomenon, owing to myriad factors potentially affecting immunogenicity. For the purposes of this book, these factors are grouped into two categories: product-specific factors such as product origin, glycosylation, aggregation, impurities and formulation, and patient-related characteristics such as genetic makeup and immune status and competency. These numerous and varied factors impose challenges to immunogenicity risk assessment and development of risk mitigation strategies. The intrinsic complexity of detection, quantification, characterization, and control or mitigation of ADA argues for advanced statistical methods in both study design and analysis. This book is intended to provide a single source of information on statistical concepts, principles, methods, and strategies for detection, quantification, assessment, and control of immunogenicity.

The book consists of six chapters. Chapter 1 provides an overview of immunogenicity, its impact on biopharmaceutical development, regulatory requirements, statistical methods and strategies used for immunogenicity detection, quantification, risk assessment, and mitigation. Chapter 2 deals with ADA assay development, optimization, validation, and transfer based on sound statistical principles, design, and analysis. It discusses statistical considerations in many aspects of screening, confirmatory, and neutralizing assay development. Chapter 3 is focused on analysis of cut point, a key assay performance parameter in ADA assay development and validation. It covers a wide range of topics from sample size calculation, data normalization, outlier detection and removal, to selection of proper models for cut point analysis. Challenges and limitations of cut point applied to practical clinical sample testing are also explained. In Chapter 4, we illustrate how to apply statistical modeling approaches to establishing associations between ADA and clinical outcomes, and process parameters, predicting immunogenicity risk, and developing risk-mitigation strategies. Various strategies for immunogenicity risk control are presented in Chapter 5. Finally, the majority of computer codes/algorithms of the statistical methods introduced in the book are provided and explained in Chapter 6.

In recent years, assessment of immunogenicity has emerged as an important regulatory initiative as evidenced by a growing number of white papers on the subject, and publication of the FDA and EMA guidelines. It is also a crucial step toward using risk-based strategies in biopharmaceutical product development. To ensure regulatory compliance, gain deep understanding of immunogenicity, and develop effective immunogenicity risk mitigation strategies, it is imperative to apply robust statistical methods and thinking in the detection, quantification, assessment, and mitigation of immunogenicity risk. To that end, a single book covering statistical concepts, principles, methods, and strategies in immunogenicity assessment will provide an invaluable resource for practitioners in biopharmaceutical therapy development. As immunogenicity risk assessment and control are issues faced by professionals who are involved in non-clinical, clinical, and bioprocess development, this book will be helpful to many individuals in various scientific and regulatory disciplines, including statisticians, pharmacokineticists, toxicologists, clinical assay developers, clinicians, biopharmaceutical engineers, and regulatory reviewers.

We are extremely grateful to John Kimmel, executive editor, Chapman & Hall/CRC Press, for giving us the opportunity to work on this book. We would like to express our gratitude to Laura Richman, Dianne Hirsch, and Kicab Castañeda-Méndez for their expert review of the book and helpful comments.

Harry Yang
Jianchun Zhang
Binbing Yu
Wei Zhao
Gaithersburg, Maryland, USA

List of Figures

List of Tables

1

Introduction

CONTENTS

1.1 Background

The discovery of DNA in 1953, and the many advances made afterwards in cellular and molecular biology in the late 1970s brought into existence the biotechnology industry. Of particular importance was the development of recombinant DNA technology which enabled the creation and production of proteins in a laboratory setting. These technological advances have provided biopharmaceutical companies with the tools needed to develop "targeted therapies" aimed at the biological underpinnings of various diseases. The first recombinant biologic therapy licensed in the United States (U.S.) was recombinant human insulin which was approved by U.S. Food and Drug Administration (FDA) in 1982. Since the approval of recombinant human insulin, more than 200 biological products have been approved over the past several decades, treating diseases ranging from cancers to rare genetic disorders (Guilford-Blake and Strickland (2008)). As of 2013, more than 900 molecules, targeting over 100 diseases including cancer, multiple sclerosis, and rheumatoid arthritis, were at various stages of development (PhRMA (2013)). These biotechnology-derived therapeutics hold a great deal of promise for future medicinal innovation and breakthroughs.

However, despite the promise of therapeutic proteins and monoclonal antibodies to meet unmet medical needs, development of biologics poses a host of unique challenges. Biopharmaceutical products are often large in size, having complex structures which are often modified post-translationally, e.g., glycosylation, and/or during manufacturing to improve product quality, e.g. pegylation. Additionally, most therapeutic proteins are produced in non-human cell lines and therefore are not identical to the homologous human protein. In light of these complexities, it is not surprising that the manufacture of biologics requires complicated and tightly controlled manufacturing processes. An additional consideration is that most biologics are administered intravenously or subcutaneously. As a result, therapeutic proteins and monoclonal antibodies (mAbs) have the potential to induce immune responses when administered to patients.

One common immunogenic response to therapeutic proteins and mAbs is the development of anti-drug antibodies (ADA). While the development of ADAs against therapeutic proteins is common and often has no measurable clinical effects, ADA responses have the potential to negatively affect both patient safety and product efficacy (Shankar et al. (2008)). For instance, for a therapeutic protein that has a non-redundant endogenous counterpart, a neutralizing antibody response can cross-react with the endogenous protein, causing serious consequences (FDA (2014)). One example is recombinant human erythropoietin (rhEPO) which is used to treat anemia. It was shown that neutralizing antibodies (NAbs) directed against rhEPO secondary to administration of the product also blocked the function of endogenous erythropoietin which was causal in the development of pure red cell aplasia (Casadevall et al. (2002)). ADA binding to the therapeutic can also impact product efficacy. For instance, 50% patients treated with the murine monoclonal antibody OKT3 developed human anti-mouse antibodies (HAMAs) that correlated with decreased efficacy (Kuus-Reichel et al. (1994)). Readers interested in reviews on immunogenicity are referred to van de Weert and Møller (2008) and Baker et al. (2010).

In recent years, various methods and strategies have been developed to reduce and manage immunogenicity of biologic products. Early efforts were centered on methods for measuring ADA. Now, in addition to ADA monitoring, therapeutic protein manufacturers are increasingly focusing on engineering therapeutics with reduced risk of inducing ADA responses. Approaches include development of humanized proteins, removal of T-cell epitopes, and selection of less immunogenic proteins using *in silico*, *in vitro*, and *in vivo* prediction methods. Therapeutic proteins are often produced in non-human cell lines and species, e.g., mice. As such, their protein sequences differ from the human counterpart, thus increasing immunogenic potential of the therapeutic protein when administered to human recipients. Humanization of proteins produced in non-human species is a process to increase the proteins similarity, through modifying non-human sequences to homologous human sequences. In certain cases, humanization has been shown to be effective in reducing the risk of immunogenicity. In one retrospective review of ADA responses to mAbs, murine mAbs were shown to have the highest frequency of ADA responses, and that replacement of the mouse immunoglobin constant regions with human sequences reduced the development of ADAs (Hwang and Foote (2005)). ADA responses to T-cell epitopes is also well recognized. It has been shown that the presence of T-cell epitopes in a therapeutic protein is one driver of ADA responses. When T-cell receptors recognize small fragments derived from protein antigens coupled with major histocompatibility complex (MHC) class II molecules on the surface of antigen-presenting cells (APCs), T-cell responses are activated. Therefore, one way to minimize immunogenic risk is to deactivate T-cell responses to a therapeutic protein. For this purpose, several methods have been utilized to identify and design proteins that have a more acceptable immunogenic profile. The strategies include removal of T-cell epitopes through *in silico*, *in vitro*, and *in vivo* prediction, patient immunosuppression and tolerization (Adair and Ozanne (2002)). Using *in-vitro* experiments, T-cell epitopes can be screened and then proteins with the least T-cell epitopes can be used for subsequent development. Immunosuppression reduces immunogenicity through treating subjects with drugs that suppress T-cell activities; whereas the tolerance approach focuses on desensitizing the immune system to the therapeutic protein so that the therapeutic protein is no longer recognized as foreign.

As pointed out by De Groot and Martin (2009), successful mitigation of immunogenicity potential of a therapy is likely to rely on a combined approach. It uses rational sequence design, and *in vitro* and *in vivo* animal testing to select the least immunogenic lead candidates to advance into clinical testing stage. Equally important is the assessment of other triggers that may cause undesirable immune responses.

It is now well understood that there are many other factors related to the product, process, and patient that may cause immunogenicity. It involves understanding the characteristics of the molecules, their intended use, factors impacting immunogenicity, development of sensitive assays for the detection, quantification, characterization of ADA, and careful design of risk-mitigation strategies. However, effective immunogenicity risk management in production and clinical development of the therapeutic proteins depends heavily on the ability to effectively synthesize and quantitatively evaluate information from multiple sources. The intrinsic complexity of quantitative evaluations argues for advanced statistical methods in both study design and analysis. In this chapter, we provide an overview of immunogenicity issues, with a focus on the development of ADAs, regulatory requirements, and strategies that can be used to mitigate immunogenicity risk. Applications of statistical concepts, principles, and methods to address immunogenicity issues are briefly described. In depth coverage of statistical methods used to evaluate immunogenicity is provided in Chapters 2-5.

1.2   Immunogenicity

Immune responses are the natural defense mechanism of vertebrates against disease causing pathogens. Immunogenicity is the ability of an antigen to elicit immune responses. There are two types of immune responses. The innate immune response is the first line of host defense against a pathogen. Activation of an innate immune response occurs by an antigen binding to germ-line encoded receptors on antigen presenting cells (APCs), such as macrophages and dendritic cells, followed by antigen internalization and degradation. Following degradation, peptide fragments are moved to the extracellular cell membrane where they form Major Histocompatibility (MHC)-peptide complexes. The cell-mediated immune system, also known as the adaptive immune system, is the second line of defense against pathogens. In the cell-mediated response, CD4+ helper T cells and CD8+ cytotoxic T cells are activated when they bind to the MHC-peptide complexes on the APCs. Activation of signaling pathways that lead to the development of anti-antigen antibodies is mediated by CD4+ T cells. In brief, cytokines released by CD4+ T cells stimulate B cells to proliferate and differentiate into plasma cells that produce antibodies specific to one of the pathogen's peptides.

Immune responses can be either wanted or unwanted. Wanted immunogenicity is the immune response against pathogens including viruses and bacteria, which is typically induced with injection of a vaccine. Unwanted immunogenicity is the immune response against a therapeutic protein, such as a monoclonal antibody, through production of ADAs. ADA responses to therapeutic proteins are a complex phenomenon, owing to myriad factors that can potentially affect immunogenicity. In general, these factors are classified into two categories: product-related and patient-related. Product-related factors that influence the development of ADA responses include species-specific epitopes, levels and types of glycosylation, levels of protein aggregates and impurities, and product formulation; patient-related characteristics encompass genetic makeup and immune status of the patient due to disease, route of administration, dosing frequency, and existence of endogenous equivalents (Shankar et al. (2007)). To fulfill the promise that the biologics offer, careful considerations need to be given to both biologics design and production.

1.3   Impact of Immunogenicity

As previously discussed, ADA responses to non-vaccine biologics have the potential to negatively affect both patient safety and product efficacy. For example, neutralizing ADAs (NAbs) can bind to the therapeutic protein, thus reducing the efficacy of the product, and it can be harmful when it cross-reacts with an endogenous counterpart of the therapeutic in patients. Examples of adverse ADA responses include autoimmune thrombocytopenia (ITP) following exposure to recombinant thrombopoietin, and pure red cell aplasia caused by antibodies to recombinant human EPO (rhEPO) that neutralize the product as well as endogenous EPO (Kromminga and Deray (2008), Kirshner (2011)). Additionally, both ADAs and NAbs may affect the pharmacokinetic properties of the drug by either increasing or decreasing product serum half-life which may require dosing modifications. These immunologically based consequences may cause drug developers to either terminate development or limit use of otherwise effective therapies. Since the impact of immunogenicity can be quite severe, regulatory agencies have provided guidelines for various aspects of immunogenicity assessment such as ADA assay development and risk factor identification. Common to all the regulatory documents is the requirement of managing immunogenicity risk using a risk-based approach, which helps develop risk management plan through a systematic method that links the extent of immunogenicity monitoring to the immunogenicity risk of the therapeutic protein under development.

1.4   Regulatory Environment and Guidelines

In recent years, assessment of immunogenicity has emerged as an important regulatory initiative as evidenced by a growing number of white papers on the subject, and publication of regulatory guidelines. Over the past decade, concerted efforts have been made by various working groups, consortiums, and regulatory bodies to gain a deep understanding of immunogenicity, establish best practices for ADA detection and characterization, and develop risk-based approaches to immunogenicity assessment and management. In 2000, the Ligand Binding Assay Bioanalytical Focus Group was formed under the auspice of the American Association of Pharmaceutical Scientists (AAPS), which was followed by the establishment of the Immunogenicity Working Group. Ever since, the group has produced several important publications on design, optimization, and validation of immunoassays and bioassays for detection of ADA, regulatory implications of immunogenicity, immunogenicity testing for non-clinical and clinical studies, and risk management.

Immunogenicity is a complex phenomenon involving multiple components of the immune system. Because multiple epitopes on the therapeutic may be immunogenic, ADA responses are polyclonal in nature and therefore ADAs and NAbs may both be present in samples. Therefore, it is challenging to attribute ADAs to one particular cause. In addition, it is equally difficult to obtain ADA positive controls, making detection and quantifications of ADAs formidable. Oftentimes, polyclonal or monoclonal ADAs are derived from animals and used as surrogate controls. However, they do not provide full representation of ADA from subjects given the therapeutic protein. Moreover, because ADA response vary from subject to subject, there is not only the lack of similarity between the positive control and test sample, but also lack of similarity among subjects. Therefore quantification of ADAs based on the dose response curve of positive controls is likely to introduce substantial biases. In 2004, the concept of a tiered assay approach to ADA detection and quantification was first introduced by Mire-Sluis et al. (2004). Centered on what is now known as the first tier screening assay, the authors discuss practical considerations of and provide recommendations for screening assay design and optimization. Subsequently the tiered approach concept was expanded by Geng et al. (2005) to explicitly include a tiered process in which all samples are tested using the screening assay, and only samples that are tested positive are further tested using the confirmatory assay to determine specific binding to the therapeutic protein. In 2007, the method was further expanded in Shankar et al. (2007) to include a third tier in which characterization of antibody isotopes and determination of their neutralizing activities is carried out on samples which are deemed positive by the confirmatory assay. Recommendations for the development of cell-based assays for the detection of neutralizing antibodies are provided in Gupta et al. (2007) for both non-clinical and clinical studies. A seminal paper by Shankar et al. (2008) suggests a more unified approach to ADA assay validation, which utilizes formal statistical experimental design and analysis for data normalization and transformation, outlier removal, cut point analysis, and assay quantification and validation. Simple but sufficiently rigorous statistical methods are discussed, with the understanding that use of more rigorous methods is advisable with the help of statistical professionals. More recently, risk-based strategies for detection and characterization of ADAs were recommended by Koren et al. (2008). The method proposes that the extent of ADA testing and characterization be results from risk-based assessments that determine the likelihood and severity of ADA responses. In general, the greater the risk is to the patient, the more testing and characterization is needed.

These collective efforts and important publications along with other research outcomes paved the way for several milestone publications of regulatory guidelines on assay development, including the draft guidelines "Guideline on Immunogenicity Assessment of Biotechnology-Derived Therapeutic Proteins" by the European Medicines Agency (EMA) Committee for Medicinal Products for Human Use (CHMP) (EMA (2007)), and the U.S. FDA "Draft Guidance for Industry: Assay Development for Immunogenicity Testing of Therapeutic Proteins" (FDA (2009)). In 2014, the FDA issued "Guidance for Industry:Immunogenicity Assessment for Therapeutic Protein Products" (FDA (2014)), recommending a risk-based approach be adopted for the evaluation and mitigation of ADA responses to therapeutic proteins. The scientific rationale of the FDA risk assessment strategy was fully expounded in three publications by FDA researchers which included discussions on clinical consequences of immune responses to protein therapeutics, impact of process-, product- and patient-related factors on immunogenicity, effects of changes in manufacturing, and the utility of animal models in assessing a products immunogenicity (Rosenberg and Worobec (2004a,b, 2005)). The guidelines released by the FDA and EMA provide the necessary framework for the development of robust immunogenicity assays and sound risk mitigation strategies for products under clinical development. Although there has been no formal regulatory guideline issued by the Japanese regulatory authorities, papers and presentations given by Japanese regulators suggest their requirements for immunogenicity testing, characterization, and risk control are consistent with those recommended by the EMA and FDA. In the following section, regulatory guidelines from various regulatory agencies are reviewed, and key recommendations highlighted.

1.4.1 FDA Guidelines

1.4.1.1 Tiered Approach to ADA Assay Development

In light of the cumulative knowledge of immunogenicity risk and recommendations in white papers published between 2004 and 2009 on ADA assay development, the 2009 FDA guidance adopts a tiered approach to ADA assay development. To start, a screening assay is used to classify samples into either a positive or negative category. Often easy to run, fast and sensitive, the assay provides an efficient way to detect potential ADA positive samples. Because the screening assay detects all antibodies against the therapeutic protein regardless of their functional impact, positive samples from the screening assay are subjected to a confirmatory assay to determine specificity of the ADAs against the therapeutic protein. The confirmed samples are further tested by a neutralizing antibody (NAb) assay to assess the neutralizing capability of the ADA against the therapeutic protein. Additionally, other tests aimed at assessing immunoglobulin subclasses or the isotypes of the ADAs and their epitope specificity, cross-reactivity with endogenous proteins, and other characteristics may also be carried out. This approach has been widely adopted by analytical laboratories that specialize in immunogenicity detection and quantification. A diagram of this tiered approach is presented in Figure 1.1.

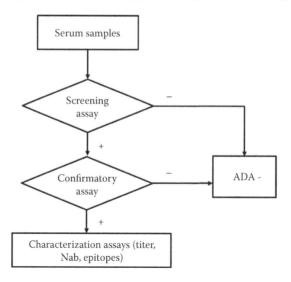

FIGURE 1.1
Tiered approach to immunogenicity assessment.

The FDA guidance points out that results of pre-clinical testing is not predictive of immunogenicity in human subjects, but acknowledges that immunogenicity from animal models may be useful for pre-clinical safety assessments, and may provide insight for the monitoring of antibody-related toxicities in human studies. The FDA guidance also allows for an evolving ADA assay development and validation paradigm that allows implementation of preliminary validated assays for use in preclinical and early clinical trials. However, results from fully validated assays are required for the licensure application.

Key parameters that need to be considered for ADA assays intended for human sample testing include: (1) Sensitivity: the assays should detect clinically meaningful levels of ADAs; (2) Interference: effects of therapeutic drug in sample and sample matrix should be evaluated; (3) Functional or physiological consequences: the assays should detect neutralizing activity of ADAs; and (4) Risk-based application: for each product, a careful sampling plan and testing strategy should be developed based on probability that product will elicit an immune response and the potential severity of the ADA response.

For assays in each of the three tiers, the FDA guidance provides ADA assay design considerations such as assay format, positive and negative controls, and minimum required dilution, cut point, matrix effect, and drug tolerance (FDA (2009)). Also suggested are key validation parameters including sensitivity, specificity, precision, robustness and stability. For all assays, the guidance recommends test samples be obtained at appropriate time points considering the product's's half-life and dosing frequency. For example, for IgM detection, it is optimal to collect samples 7-14 days after exposure whereas samples taken at 4-6 weeks post treatment are recommended for determining IgG responses. It is also recommended to collect pre-exposure samples that can be tested, and used as baseline measures for assessing drug-related ADA responses.

1.4.1.2 Immunogenicity Risk Assessment

In August 2014, the U.S. FDA published a guidance entitled "Guidance for Industry: Immunogenicity Assessment for Therapeutic Protein Products." Recognizing the immunogenic potential of biologics that may adversely impact patient safety and product efficacy, the guideline recommends a risk-based approach to mitigating immunogenicity risk. Central to this approach is a thorough understanding of clinical consequences of ADA responses, identification of factors that may affect the immunogenicity of the product under development, and development of risk control strategies. To that end, the guidance describes various product- and patient-specific factors that have the potential to affect the immunogenicity of protein therapeutics and provides detailed recommendations pertaining to each of these factors that may reduce the likelihood of unwanted immune responses. Furthermore, the guidance affords a series of risk mitigation strategies which can be employed in the clinical development of protein therapeutics. In addition, supplemental information on the diagnosis and management of particular adverse consequences of immune responses is provided, along with discussions of the uses of animal studies, and the conduct of comparative immunogenicity studies.

Clinical Consequences

As stated in the FDA guidances, administration of therapeutic protein products in patients often results in unwanted immune responses of varying clinical relevance. Adverse events may range from transient antibody responses with no apparent clinical manifestations to life-threatening and catastrophic reactions. To mitigate such risk, it is imperative to understand the underlying immunologic mechanism, and devise risk control strategies accordingly.

Impact on Efficacy

Development of both neutralizing and non-neutralizing antibodies as a result of immunogenicity can cause loss of efficacy in product recipients. This is of particular concern when the product is a life-saving therapeutic. For example, persistent ADAs to the treatments of metabolic diseases may complicate the intervention, resulting in diminished clinical benefits, disease progression, and even death. Less severe consequences include alteration of the pharmacokinetic profile of the product, which may require dose modifications. In addition, ADAs may have an impact on pharmacodynamics by misdirecting the therapeutic protein to target Fc Receptor (FcR) bearing cells, thereby reducing efficacy. Therefore, the FDA guidance recommends determining the clinical relevance of both binding and neutralizing antibody responses by correlating them with clinical manifestations.

Consequences for Safety

As previously discussed, the safety consequences of immunogenicity are wide-ranged. Although ADA responses often do not cause adverse events, some incidences of ADA-induced adverse events have been observed. The guideline outlines major safety concerns associated with immunogenicity. They include acute allergic reactions such as anaphylaxis. However, it is recognized in the guidance that the presence of ADA alone is not necessarily predictive of anaphylaxis or other hypersensitivity reactions. The clinical relevance of these ADAs can only be elucidated through correlation with clinical responses. This is a subject that is studied at length in Chapter 4. Other safety concerns comprise cytokine release syndrome(CRS) caused by the rapid release of pro-inflammatory cytokines, infusion reactions ranging from discomfort to severe reactions, non-acute reactions such as delayed hypersensitivity, and finally, in cases where the products have endogenous counterparts critical for certain physiological functions, cross-reactivity to endogenous proteins.

Factors Affecting Immunogenicity

Immunogenicity is a complex phenomenon, owing to myriad factors potentially affecting immunogenicity. The risk factors can be categorized into patient-specific factors such as genetic makeup and immune status of the patient and product-specific characteristics of which some are product-intrinsic such as glycosylation, aggregation, impurities and formulation and others are product-extrinsic factors including route of administration, dosing frequency, and existence of endogenous equivalents. Understanding of these risk factors is the foundation for the development of effective risk mitigation strategies for unwanted immunogenicity. For example, murine mAbs are known to elicit immunogenicity. Recent technology advances make possible replacement of murine amino acid sequences with human sequences. As such, there has been notable decline of immunogenicity incidences due to use of humanized mAbs. However, despite the progress, immunogenicity issues persist even for therapies of humanized mAbs. It is critical to approach immunogenicity risk control from a holistic perspective, which includes identification of risk factors and development of risk-mitigating strategies.

- Patient-Specific Factors

  Certain patient's characteristics may predispose the subjects to the development of undesirable immunogenic reactions to some products. For example, patients with an activated immune system due to certain infections or autoimmune disease may have high chances to mount immune responses to therapeutic product than those whose immune systems are compromised. Other factors include the patient's age, genetic makeup. The guidance emphasizes the need for the manufacturer to provide a clear rationale to support the selection of an appropriate study population, especially for first-in-human studies. Additional risk factors include sensitization of patient's prior exposure to the drug or similar protein, and/or to the excipients, and/or process/product-related impurities; route, dose, and frequency of administration; patient's genetic makeup and status of tolerance to the homologous endogenous proteins. Table 1.1 summarizes patient-specific factors along with risk control recommendation in the FDA guidance.

TABLE 1.1

Patient-specific factors that affect immunogenicity and risk-mitigating strategies

Factors	Recommendation
Immunologic Status and Competency	Provide a rationale to support selection of study population, especially for first-in-human studies
Prior Sensitization	Screen for history of relevant allergies. Dosing based on individual risk-benefit assessment
Route of Administration, Dose, and Frequency	Carefully select route of administration
Genetic Status	Evaluate genetic factors to predispose patients to ADA development
Tolerance to Endogenous Protein	Gain robust understanding of immune tolerance to endogenous protein

- Product-Specific Factors

  The FDA guidance also lists nine product-intrinsic factors that may affect immunogenicity. They include product origin, structural and functional characteristics of the product such as presence of aggregates, glycosylation and pegylation variants. Detailed discussion of the impact of these factors may have on the product can be found in the guidance. The factors are listed in Table 1.2, with corresponding recommendations of risk management.

TABLE 1.2
Product-specific factors that affect immunogenicity and risk-mitigating strategies

Factors	Recommendation
Product Origin	Naturally sourced products should be evaluated for other protein and non-protein components
Prior Structure and Post Translational Modification	For fusion molecules, studies to define antigenic site of antibody response are recommended
Aggregates	Minimize protein aggregation to the maximal extent possible
Glycosylation/Pegylation	Use proper cell substrate production system that glycosylates the therapeutic protein in a nonimmunogenic manner. Assays for antibodies to PEG itself should be developed and utilized
Impurities with Adjuvant Activity	Use assays of high sensitivity and clinical relevance to detect and quantitate levels of innate immune response modulating impurities
Immunomodulatory Properties	Monitor product potential for autoimmunity from the earliest stages of product development
Formulation	Evaluate excipients for potential to prevent product denaturation and degradation
Container Closure	Test for leachables on product under both stress and real-time storage conditions
Product Custody	Educate patients. Ensure cold chain security

A Risk-Based Strategy

A risk-based approach to immunogenicity assessment is recommended in the FDA guidances. The method consists of assessments of the overall risk of the therapeutic protein, identification of risk factors, and development of control strategies, which includes a risk management plan for clinical testing, and measures to minimize chances of unwanted immune responses. In general, the greater the immunogenicity potential the protein has, the more stringent the risk management plan should be. The risk-based approach lends drug developers the tools for development of therapeutics, in the presence of potential immunogenicity risk.

1.4.2 European Medicines Agency (EMA) Guidance

1.4.2.1 EMA Guidelines on Immunogenicity Assessment

In 2007, EMA released a draft guideline entitled "Immunogenicity Assessment of Biotechnology-Derived Therapeutic Proteins" (EMA (2007)). The scope of the guideline covers proteins and polypeptides, their derivatives, and products of which they are components, for example, conjugates. These proteins and polypeptides are primarily derived from recombinant or non-recombinant expression systems. General recommendations and principles are provided to guide developers and assessors on immunogenicity evaluation. The guideline discusses factors that may affect immunogenic responses, utilities of non-clinical assessment of immunogenicity, development of analytical methods for detecting and quantifying ADAs in clinical samples, potential clinical consequences of immunogenicity, immunogenicity and clinical development, and immunogenicity risk management plans.

The EMA 2007 guideline stresses that therapeutic proteins should be seen as individual products, and experience from related proteins can only be considered supportive. Therefore, immunogenicity evaluation needs to be studied for each product and each indication/patient population. The guideline also classifies risk factors into patient- and disease-related, and product- and process-related characteristics which are similar to the lists provided in Tables 1.1 and 1.2. Patient-related factors include genetic factors that are either modulating the immune response or related to a gene defect, age, disease-related factors (severity and stage of a disease), concomitant treatment(s), duration of and route of administration, treatment modalities, and previous exposure to similar or related proteins. Product factors that may influence the immunogenic potential of the therapeutic are the origin and nature of the related/similar protein (structural homology, post-translational modifications), modification of the native protein (e.g. pegylation), product- and process-related impurities (e.g. breakdown products, aggregates and host cell proteins, lipids or DNA), and formulation.

Like the FDA guidance, the EMA document indicates that there is limited utility in using results of non-clinical studies to predict immunogenicity in human. However, animal models can be used to compare immunogenicity responses for similar biological products, and for changes to the manufacturing process. The EMA guideline also recommends a tiered approach to the development of reliable and robust methods for immunogenicity assessment. The guideline also stresses that careful consideration should be given to sampling schedule for immunogenicity assessment in clinical trials, and inclusion of all patients for such assessment. For the market authorization application, an immunogenicity risk management plan is required. Post-marketing studies may be needed to further evaluate the product immunogenic potential.

Subsequent to the 2007 EMA guideline, EMA issued a guideline entitled "Guideline on Immunogenicity Assessment of Monoclonal Antibodies Intended for In Vivo Clinical Use," which came into effect in December, 2012.

This guideline addresses immunogenicity issues of mAbs intended for clinical use. Once again, a risk-based approach is recommended. The guideline includes assessments of risk factors impacting immunogenicity of mAbs, clinical consequences, and considerations in ADA assay development, in particular, for neutralizing antibodies.

Two additional EMA guidelines, which discuss immunogenicity issues, were released in 2012 and 2013. One is a guideline on similar biological medicinal products containing mAbs (EMA (2013)) and the other on similar biological medicinal products containing biotechnology-derived proteins as the active substance (EMA (2012)). Both guidelines recommend comparability immunogenicity assessments between the innovator drug and biosimilar version of the drug. It is further recommended that the innovator therapeutic protein and the biosimilar product be tested using the same validated ADA assays. In instances when the biosimilar product has a higher level or frequency of immunogenicity than the innovator biologic, a comparison of risk to benefit may be necessary. In addition, long-term immunogenicity data post-authorization might be required especially in cases where the duration of comparability study included in the licensure application was short.

1.4.2.2 Latest Development of EMA Immunogenicity Guidelines

Since the publications of 2007 and 2009 EMA guidelines, a considerable amount of information and knowledge has been gained concerning ADA assays, risk factors, and clinical consequences of immunogenicity including loss of efficacy, hypersensitivity, and cross-reactivity with endogenous proteins. In consideration of these cumulative knowledge and issues observed in assessment of market authorization applications (MAAs), in March 2014, the EMA published a concept paper, announcing its intent to revise the 2007 guideline. The revision will address issues including: (1) More specific guidance for the presentation of immunogenicity data; (2) Requirements of data on antibody assays; (3) Role of *in vitro* and *in vivo* non-clinical studies; (4) Risk-based approaches to immunogenicity; (5) Clinical data to study the correlations of the induced antibodies to allergic and anaphylactic/anaphylactoid reactions, delayed immunological reactions, pharmacokinetics, lack of efficacy; (6) Comparative immunogenicity studies; and (7) Post-licensing immunological studies. The EMA stated that the aim of the revision is not to increase the number of studies on immunogenicity, but to increase the quality of the studies and their clarity to the assessors.

1.4.3 Japanese Regulatory Requirements of Immunogenicity

So far, there have been no formal regulatory documents issued by the Japanese regulatory authorities. However, the agency fully recognizes that immunogenicity is a critical issue in the manufacture, clinical, and commercial use of the therapeutic proteins (Hayakawa and Ishii-Watabe (2011)). Since the middle of 1980s, many biological products have been approved in Japan. Drawing from the experience and knowledge gained from those approvals, the Japanese regulatory authority requires immunogenicity be tested in both non-clinical and clinical studies. They also suggest mitigating immunogenicity risk using risk-minimizing approaches, which include reducing product- and process-related risk factors and management of treatments with known risk. For example, *in silico* studies can be carried out to help select candidate sequences that are less immunogenic, and biomarker studies can be used exclude high-risk patients from clinical trials. The Japanese regulatory authority also acknowledges that, in the long run, advances in *in silico* technology and development of more relevant animal models will doubtlessly help select less immunogenic proteins for clinical development. However, in the short term, pre-approval data including those from both nonclinical and clinical studies might not be sufficient to gain an adequate understanding of product immunogenic profiles. Firms have to rely on post-approval surveillance programs to gain a solid understanding of the product immunogenicity risk. In principle, similar to the U.S FDA and the EMA, the Japanese regulatory authority advocates a risk-based approach to immunogenicity assessment.

1.5 Statistics in Immunogenicity Risk Assessment

All biologics become potentially immunogenic under specific circumstances. The risk varies considerably among products, patient populations, and treatment regimens. In general, a risk-based approach to assessing immunogenicity is recommended by regulatory guidelines and has been widely adopted by drug manufacturers and clinical investigators. The method is developed on a case-by-case basis. As pointed out by Koren et al. (2008), the essential components of a risk-based approach to immunogenicity assessment include (1) understanding molecular characteristics of the therapeutic protein; (2) its mechanism of action (MOA) and intended use; (3) target population; (4) risk factors that were discussed in the previous section; (5) associated risk control strategies. The knowledge of the protein's molecular characteristics, MOA, therapeutic indication, and intended recipients helps classify the molecule into different risk categories such as low, moderate, or high risk. These classifications will impact the ADA testing plan including sampling time and frequency during clinical development. For example, the more immunogenic the molecule is, the more frequent the ADA testing needs to be conducted. It is also essential to identify risk factors through an objective risk assessment, based on prior knowledge and historical data. For this purpose, laboratory, nonclinical data, and clinical experience can be utilized. Once the risk factors are identified and risk level determined, proper control strategies can be devised.

Virtually all aspects of immunogenicity risk assessment involve applications of statistical methods and principles. The unique challenges of predicting immunogenicity either *in silico*, *in vitro* or *in vivo* in animal models, developing sensitive and reliable ADA assays in the absence of reference standards, establishing ADA association with clinical sequelae, identifying risk factors, and devising immunogenicity risk-mitigating strategies require the application of advanced statistical methods. For example, since there are usually multiple factors that contribute to risk of immunogenicity, risk assessment needs to be conducted in a holistic manner. Multivariate analyses, which account for interdependence among potential risk factors, and time-dependent nature of ADA measurements collected at different sampling points, are likely to be effective tools for exploring association of ADAs with the various risk factors described in the introduction. In addition, understanding that the sample sizes might be small and incidence of ADA might be low for some early studies, mixture models or meta-analysis might be explored to describe the associations.

1.5.1   *In Silico* Prediction of Immunogenicity

A brief synopsis of the roles of MHC molecules in regulating T-cell responses, which are well characterized, are briefly explained here. MHC molecules bind to peptides which are expressed of the surface of APCs and which are recognizable by T-cell receptor, thus activating T-cell responses. In recent years, *in silico* methods have been developed to identify peptides which may have high affinity to the MHC binding grove, which could trigger strong immune responses. Since the binding grove of MHC class I molecules are closed at both ends, the sizes of peptide sequences that bind to this class of molecules are short, and it is relatively easy to predict their affinity to MHC-I molecules. By contrast, the binding groove of MHC Class II molecules are open at both ends. As a consequence, peptides of varying lengths can bind to the MHC Class II groove. While useful in rational design of therapeutic proteins, prediction of MHC Class II binding peptides is much more challenging. Research of binding motifs revealed that a segment of nine amino acids within a peptide is instrumental in peptide-MHC-binding (Zhang et al. (2008)). Computer algorithms based on various statistical modeling methods such as artificial neural network and Gibbs sampling can be used to predict MHC-II-binding peptides (Brusic et al. (1998), Nielsen et al. (2004)).

1.5.2   ADA Detection and Quantification

Key to successful evaluation of immunogenicity is to have well developed, validated, and sensitive assays. Such assays enable objective detection and characterization of ADAs, and render confidence in the data used for immunogenicity assessment. However, there are many challenges associated with ADA assay development, optimization, and validation. For example, lack of reference standards makes it extremely hard to accurately estimate an ADA assay detection limit (Dodge et al. (2009)). Furthermore, although various assay platforms such as enzyme-linked immunosorbent assay (ELISA) and electrochemiluminescene-based assay (ECLA) are well understood scientifically and several guidelines are available for ADA assay development and validation (FDA (2009), Mire-Sluis et al. (2004), Shankar et al. (2008)), data analysis and interpretation has become increasingly sophisticated and remains challenging. While the published works (e.g., Shankar et al. (2008)) cover a broad array of statistical issues related to ADA assay development, they fall short on development of effective statistical methods to solve the problems (Zhang et al. (2013)). For example, Kubiak et al. (2013) demonstrated that the results from screening assays and confirmatory assays are highly correlated. Yet, there has been no method developed so far that can effectively account for such correlations. As a result, estimated false-positive rates are likely inflated. Likewise, for sample size determination, cut point analysis, outlier removal, comparison between sample populations from validation and in-study experiments, utility of tiered approach, and overall reporting of ADA results all need careful scientific and statistical evaluations (Zhang et al. (2013), Zhang et al. (2014), Gorovits (2009)). In addition, because ADA assays are often developed under stringent timeline, utilization of statistical design of experiment (DOE) strategies is advantageous in understanding the effects of multiple factors and their interaction on ADA assay performance (Ray et al. (2009)).

1.5.3 Clinical Characterization of ADA

As previously discussed, clinical consequences of immunogenic response comprise altered exposure to the drug, compromised efficacy, and adverse events ranging from transient appearance of ADAs to severe life-threatening reactions. It is critically important to assess the impact of ADA on the efficacy and safety of the therapeutic protein. The ADA responses also need to be further correlated with parameters such as pharmacokinetics and pharmacodynamics to gain a deeper understanding of the clinical effects of ADA (Wadhwa et al. (2003)). Efforts have been made to develop a harmonized strategy for the assessment and reporting of data from clinical immunogenicity studies of therapeutic proteins and peptides (Shankar et al. (2014)). This approach has the potential to maximize the utility of immunogenicity data from clinical trials. Three aspects of ADAs are of particularly interest, and are recommended to be reported. They include (1) characteristics of ADA reactions; (2) relationships of ADAs with clinical pharmacokinetics (PK) and pharmacodynamics (PD); and (3) relationships of ADAs with clinical safety and efficacy.

1.5.3.1 Characteristics of ADA Immune Response

The ADA incidence rate is a key measure of immunogenic response. Accurate estimation of ADA responses helps assess the immunogenic potential of the therapeutic protein. ADA can be characterized through many clinical endpoints such as number of ADA incidences within a fixed observational time, probability of occurrence, and time to first detection of ADAs. Statistical methods that provide estimation of these endpoints are discussed in Chapter 4.

1.5.3.2 Correlation between ADA and PK/PD, Clinical Safety and Efficacy

ADAs induced by administration of protein therapeutics has an impact on their PK/PD characteristics. ADAs with high affinities for the protein therapeutic have an increased likelihood of modulating and even neutralizing the drugs therapeutic effects. For example, drug-clearing or drug-sustaining ADA responses can cause increased or decreased drug clearance rates, respectively, thus necessitating dose modifications. The characterization of these ADA responses presents experimental challenges because of many technological limitations including inability to measure absolute ADA concentration or affinity. For example, ADA responses may not correlate well with the true immune response as they vary when different assay platforms are used. Mathematical models incorporating PK/PD and ADA features can provide significant insights which can be used to characterize ADA responses such as severity of the response, and the elimination rate of ADA-drug complexes. Discussions of these models are provided in Chapter 4. In addition, traditional statistical models such as fixed, mixed effects, and/or repeated measurement models can be used to assess the impact of ADA frequency, time to first ADA episode, duration of ADA on PK/PD parameters/profiles. Bayesian analysis may also be utilized to differentiate PK/PD profiles between ADA-positive and -negative subjects.

1.5.3.3 Relationship of ADA with Clinical Efficacy and Safety

The correlation of ADA characteristics, in terms of magnitude, frequency, and duration, with clinical endpoints can be modeled within a multivariate framework. Multivariate approaches which accommodate inter-dependence among response variables may enhance the detectability of statistical significant associations. These approaches are particularly useful when data are limited.

1.5.3.4 Identification of Risk Factors

Identification of risk factor starts with the determination of the criticality of each factor. The criticality of a factor is determined based on the impact immunogenicity has on product safety and efficacy. The criticality of a factor can usually be determined through a risk assessment process. As the first step, the assessment determines both the severity of immunogenicity due to the risk factor and the probability or likelihood for the immunogenic event to occur. The severity ranks the risk factor based on the consequences of the immunogenic reaction; whereas, likelihood of the immunogenic event characterizes the probability for an immunogenic event to occur when the risk factor is outside of its acceptable range. The determination of both severity and likelihood requires knowledge of both the product and process, and depends heavily on laboratory, non-clinical, and clinical data. Statistical tools ranging from graphical displays to sophisticated modeling are important in the identification of risk factors.

1.5.4 Control of Immunogenicity Risk

Although general strategies for immunogenicity risk control have been discussed in the literature and outlined in regulatory guidelines, the control strategies are product-dependent. In addition, as immunogenicity is impacted by so many risk factors which are usually correlated and interdependent, it is important to account for their joint effects in the design of risk mitigation strategies. In this regard, two methods are of particular interest. One is to reduce immunogenicity risk due to process- and product-related factors through setting appropriate acceptance ranges for the critical factors predicted to be involved in the development of immunogenicity. The other concerns segmenting the patient population so as to identify a subset of the population that has less potential to have immune response to the treatment. Such a subset can be used as the target population for the clinical development of the therapeutic protein.

1.5.4.1 Control of Process/Product Factors

Product- and process- related factors are often involved in the development of immunogenicity. Oftentimes, these risk factors are correlated, and have a joint impact on immunogenicity. For example, aggregation is frequently identified as a risk factor of great concern. However, the immunogenic potential of aggregation is likely dependent on the mechanism of action of the therapeutic protein. It may or may not have a significant impact depending on the nature of the target molecule (immunostimulatory or immunomodulatory). By identifying critical risk factors and controlling them jointly within ranges such that movement within the ranges would not cause immunogenicity concerns. Clinical data with measurements of risk factors and immunogenicity incidences are most useful in establishing the acceptance ranges. Statistical models can be used to link the risk factors to the ADA incidences, thus enabling acceptance criteria to be set in a clinical meaningful fashion. More discussion on this subject is given in Chapter 5.

1.5.4.2 Biomarkers for Immunogenicity

As previously discussed, some patient's characteristics predispose the subject to have an immunogenic response to the biological therapies. One way to mitigate this immunogenic risk is to segment the patient population so that a subset of the population that is less likely to have immune reaction is identified. This subpopulation will be the target population for the biologic clinical development. In the literature, some markers are used to indicate possible immunogenicity. For example, usually high and persisting levels of neutralizing antibodies are indicative of immunogenicity (Cornips and Schellekens (2010)), and can be potentially used to exclude high risk patients from enrolling into clinical studies. However, since factors that impact immunogenicity are rarely independent, the use of a univariate marker is inadequate to differentiate one group of subjects from another. In Chapter 5, various statistical methods for patient segmentation and biomarker discovery are introduced. They include cluster analysis, principal component analysis, and predictive modeling based on discriminant analysis. These methods are illustrated using simulated examples.

1.6 Statistical Considerations in Comparative Immunogenicity Studies

Immunogenicity issues can also arise in the development of biosimilar products. Although the follow-on biologic might be derived from the same substrate as the reference product, the raw materials might be from different sources and there might be differences in manufacturing process that can potentially increase the risk of immunogenicity. In the EMA guideline on "Similar Biological Medicinal Products Containing Biotechnology-Derived Proteins as Active Substance: Non-Clinical and Clinical Issues," (EMA (2013)) it is stated that immunogenicity testing of the biosimilar and the reference products should be conducted within the comparability exercise by using the same assay format and sampling schedule. Assays should be performed with both the reference and biosimilar molecules in parallel (in a blinded fashion) to measure the immune response against the product that was received by each patient. Therefore, a formal immunogenicity study is required to establish comparable immunogenicity profiles between the biosimilar and reference product. The study needs to be carefully planned, sample size adequately determined, and sample testing scheme well thought out to ensure collection of sufficient and quality data. Several study design considerations are discussed in Chow (2013). They include patient population, randomization, and washout period for cross-over design, inter- and intra-product variability, sample size, and surrogate endpoints. Various methods for sample size calculations are provided. As comparative immunogenicity study design and analysis is beyond the scope of this book, readers who are interested in the topic should refer to Chow (2013).

1.7 Concluding Remarks

Immunogenicity is a critical issue in the development of biologics. If not managed well, it may cause either early termination or limited use of the products. Therefore immunogenicity is a potential barrier to further development of otherwise effective treatments. Assessment and management of immunogenicity risk is a regulatory requirement and demands careful scientific, regulatory, and statistical considerations. When effectively utilized, statistical methods can be advantageous in addressing issues related to ADA assay development, risk factor identification, and development of effective control strategies. It is also worth pointing out that immunogenicity risk assessment requires expertise from various disciplines. Only through collective efforts of individuals from various scientific and regulatory disciplines, including statisticians, pharmacokineticists, toxicologists, clinical assay developers, clinicians, biopharmaceutical engineers, and regulatory reviewers, can immunogenicity issues be adequately addressed.

2

ADA Assay Development and Validation

CONTENTS

2.1   ADA Assays

The assessment of immunogenicity depends on appropriate detection, quantification, and characterization of ADAs. However, there are multiple challenges for successfully developing ADA assays. Unlike biological assays for measuring drug concentration or protein concentration in human serum, concentrations of ADAs are very low and often in magnitude of ng/mL. Due to the heterogeneity of patient characteristics and multiple epitopes on biotherapeutics,

ADA responses are likely to vary from patient to patient and change during the course of treatment. For instance, immunogenic responses can develop against epitopes previously not immunogenic. In addition, various factors such as the presence of circulating drug and concomitant drug adminstration make accurate detection of ADA even more difficult.

2.1.1 Multi-Tiered Approach

Depending on the assay signal readouts, assays typically fall into one of the following four categories: definitive quantitative, relative quantitative, quasi-quantitative, and qualitative (Lee et al. (2003)). Definitive and relative quantitative assays are those where the signal readouts having a continuous relationship with the concentration of the analyte. These assays typically have a reference standard. Concentrations of testing samples are obtained through calibration from the standard curve of the reference standard. In contrast, quasi-quantitative assays do not have reference standards and thus calibration is either not used or should be interpreted cautiously. Unlike quasi-quantitative results which are also expressed in continuous units or counts, qualitative assays generate data which take nominal values such as positive/negative or discrete values such as ordinal scores. The immunoassays for the detection and measurement of ADAs are quasi-quantitative assays, due to the lack of truly ADA positive human samples at the time of assay development and validation. Therefore, it is impossible to interpolate ADA concentration as is done for measuring drug concentration with pharmacokinetic immunoassays. As mentioned earlier, immune responses are of a rather complex nature. Therefore, a straightforward method is not available for ADA detection and characterization. Based on the many years of experimentation in the biopharmaceutical industry, it is generally accepted that a multi-tiered approach works well for ADA assays. Since then, several regulatory guidances (FDA (2009), EMA (2007), USP<1106>) and industry white papers (Mire-Sluis et al. (2004), Shankar et al. (2008), Gupta et al. (2007), Gupta et al. (2011)) regarding immunogenicity assay development and validation have been published. The multi-tiered approach is depicted in Figure 1.1 (see page 8).

In the first tier, samples are tested in a screening assay. The assay responses of these samples are compared with a threshold (cut point). Samples tested as ADA negative are not subject to further testing. If samples are tested as potentially positive, these samples are further tested in the confirmatory assay. The confirmatory assay, as a second tier is designed to confirm the specificity of potential ADA positive samples and eliminate false positive samples detected in the screening assay. The third tier of testing consists of further characterization of immune response, such as ADA titer, neutralizing activity, isotype, etc.

2.1.1.1 Screening Assay

Screening assays serve as the first step in the immunogenicity testing. They allow rapid testing of clinical trial samples. The screening assays allow a certain number of false positive samples due to the nature of complex antibody-binding. Immunoassays used for ADA detection generally are quasi-quantitative because it is not possible to generate genuine human-specific ADAs as calibrators or positive controls at the time of assay development and validation. Instead, hyperimmune serum from animals immunized with the protein therapeutic often serve as surrogates for positive controls. However, it is well known that these surrogate drug-induced ADAs generally cannot represent the human-specific ADAs. In addition, different hyperimmunized surrogate ADAs usually have different binding affinities and thus any analysis results cannot directly extrapolate to results of human population.

During the screening testing, sample immune responses are compared against a screening cut point. The screening cut point of an immunogenicity assay is the level of immune response readout in the screening assay at and above which the sample is deemed to be potentially positive for the presence of ADAs. Samples with responses below the screening cut point are declared negative and excluded from further testing. Samples with immune responses at or above the screening cut point are declared potentially positive and directed for additional testing in a confirmatory assay. Since samples below the screening cut point are not tested further, it is important to minimize false negative results. Therefore, selection of an appropriate screening cut point involves a tradeoff between false-positive and false-negative classifications. From a risk-based perspective, it is appropriate to have more false positives than false negatives during the initial screening step. Regulatory agencies and white papers recommend setting the screening cut point to allow 5% of false positive classifications. To maintain the desired false positive rate, the screening cut point is usually established using an appropriate statistical method on the data generated from individual samples. Chapter 3 is devoted to detailing various statistical methods for determining cut points.

2.1.1.2 Confirmatory Assay

Samples that are potentially positive in the screening assay are confirmed in the second tier of immunogenicity testing. The confirmatory assay is usually the same as that used for the screening assay with the exception that excess labeled soluable drug is added. By competing with a labeled drug in the screening assay, immune responses generated by ADA should be inhibited by addition of the drug, while immune responses from non-specific binding should not be inhibited or inhibited to a lesser degree. False positive samples detected in the screening step are expected to be ruled out in the confirmatory assay. As with the screening assay, a confirmatory cut point is established using statistical methods. The confirmatory cut point value of an assay is the minimum level of inhibition of a positive samples response in the presence of excess drug that determines whether the samples response is specific to the drug. Drug-specific ADA is expected to produce high inhibition and thus should be greater than a confirmatory cut point. Samples with inhibition lower than the confirmed cut point are declared negative. If samples are positive, further characterization may be necessary.

2.1.1.3   Neutralizing Assay

As mentioned before, neutralizing antibodies (NAbs) can block the biological activity of the drug and potentially impact clinical efficacy. One way that NAbs interfere with the binding of the drug to its target is by sequestering the therapeutic from its intended target and thus preventing the drug from eliciting the desired pharmacological effect. When the biotherapeutic drug has non-redundant endogenous counterpart in the human body, the NAbs are a great concern to the patient safety. Therefore, depending on the ADA incidence rate as well as the risk of the biotherapeutic drug, it is sometimes necessary to investigate the neutralizing activity of the confirmed ADA-positive samples. The neutralizing effect of NAbs can be detected using cell-based assays which best mimic the *in vivo* biological activity. Therefore, it is a regulatory expectation that cell-based assays will be used for NAb detection whenever possible. However, cell-based assays can prove extremely challenging due to a lack of appropriate cell lines and difficulties associated with their growth and maintenance. In addition, cell-based assays often suffer from low sensitivity, high variability, poor tolerance to the presence of the drug in the samples and very narrow dynamic ranges. Alternatively, ligand-binding assays can be used to analyze NAbs and are not subject to the shortcomings of cell-based assays.

2.1.2   Assay Platforms

An analytical platform utilizes certain unique physicochemical properties of the analyte of interest in order to detect and quantitate it in a matrix. A thorough understanding of these properties is indispensable to properly interpret resulting bioanalytical data. Currently, the ligand-binding assays (LBAs) are widely used for immunogenicity testing. LBAs depend on interactions between a receptor and its ligand. These interactions are characterized by high affinity and specificity. These properties make ligand-binding assays ideal for detection and quantification of biological molecules in complex matrices. Generally, in the screening step, the therapeutic protein is immobilized onto a solid support such as microtiter plate or beads. Immobilization of the therapeutic is accomplished by labeling the therapeutic protein with biotin and the solid support with either streptavidin or avidin. Because of the high affinity between biotin and streptavidin/avidin, the therapeutic protein is retained on the support matrix. If ADA molecules exist, the ADA molecules will bind to the immobilized drug proteins. The captured ADAs are then detected using another labeled reagent or drug protein. In bridged enzyme-linked immunosorbent assays (ELISAs), a signal is generated by labeling the drug with enzymes that generate colorimetric readouts. In electrochemiluminescence immunoassays, the drug is labeled with a ruthenium complex that generates light upon application of an electric current to the solid surface on which the ADA-drug complex is captured (see Figure 2.1 for a bridging assay format). One shortcoming of these assays is that the labeling and coating can block the epitopes of the therapeutic drug from binding to the ADAs, leading to potential false negatives. It is therefore important to optimize the assay for drug concentration and labeling ratios. In all, a solid understanding of advantages and limitations of the assay format can aid in the design of immunogenicity assessment program and interpretation of the resulting data. The most common formats for immunogenicity assays are briefly described below.

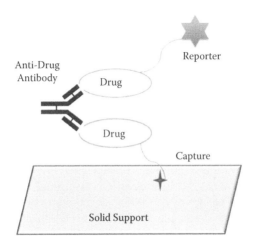

FIGURE 2.1
Schematic of bridging assay format.

Bridging assays are arguably the most common immunogenicity assay format. It depends on the ability of ADA molecules to bind more than one molecule of the drug at the same time. Two different forms of the drug are needed for the assay: one that allows ADAs to be captured onto solid surfaces and one that can serve as a reporter for generation of a signal. Upon binding of the ADAs with the two different forms of the drug, the resulting antibody-drug complex can be easily detected. Bridging assays are widely used due to their high sensitivity and capability to detect all immunoglobulin subclasses and most isotypes. Additionally, these assays can be easily applied for detection of ADAs from different species which allows use of the same format for non-clinical and clinical samples. The major disadvantage of this format is that it does not detect antibodies directly; rather, multivalent entities are capable of binding more than one molecule of the drug at the same time. For example, when the drug target is a soluble oligomer, for example, members of the tumor necrosis factor (TNF) family, it may be difficult to eliminate false positive responses.

In contrast to the bridging assays that utilizes the multivalent nature of ADAs, the direct format explicitly detects ADAs. In its simplest form, the drug is captured on a solid surface and allowed to bind ADA present in the sample. In turn, ADA is detected by using an anti-IgG antibody labeled with a reporter molecule. Direct formats suffer from two major drawbacks. First, they are not well suited for mAbs. Second, due to vast heterogeneity of ADA, the subclasses (e.g. IgG, IgM, IgE) are hard to detect.

In addition to ELISA and ECLA, there are some other platforms which have been used for immunogenicity testing. The advantages and limitations of each format and platform are summarized in Mire-Sluis et al. (2004), Parish et al. (2009), USP<1106>.

2.2   Assay Development and Validation

A reliable and reproducible immunogenicity assay is critical to the detection, quantitation and characterization of ADAs and immunogenicity assessment. Also, it is a regulatory obligation as well as of scientific interest to have a well developed and validated immunogenicity assay for its intended purpose. During assay development, various questions regarding the analytical objectives and challenges (Geng et al. (2005)) of the assay need to be asked and addressed. Appropriate assay platform is then chosen as part of the assay system which includes the selection of assay matrix, reagents and the identification of assay performance parameters. Given all these considerations, extensive efforts are needed to determine the final format and design of the assay procedure. The assay then needs to be optimized for input variables which are subject to variations. In this stage, design of experiment (DOE) methods are particularly useful to find the optimal combinations of the various assay conditions such as minimal required dilution(MRD), reagent concentration, temperature, incubation time, number of wash steps and freeze-thaw cycles, to mention a few. Once the assay is optimized, rigorous pre-study validation needs to be carried out. According to FDA guidance (FDA (2013)), "validation involves documenting, through the use of specific laboratory investigations, that the performance characteristics of a method are suitable and reliable for the intended analytical applications." A standard operating procedure(SOP) is recommended for the intended purpose with detailed description of the analytical procedure and related reagents, controls, and equipment needed to run the assay. The validation protocol should also specify assay performance parameters to be evaluated and set (or confirm) the acceptance criteria for the in-study runs. When the validation is completed, a validation report needs to be created with all the validation data and results from all assay performance parameters. In the rest of this section, several assay performance parameters are introduced with the focus on the relevant statistical methods used to analyze the parameters. In section 2.3, statistical experimental designs will be introduced with an illustration. In section 2.4, statistical methods related to assay transfer are discussed.

2.2.1 Assay Parameters

2.2.1.1 Cut Point

As explained in Shankar et al. (2008) and USP<1106>, because of the quasi-quantitative nature of ADA assay signal, it is now a routine practice to use statistical method to determine a cut point (or threshold) to classify a sample as positive or negative in immunogenicity assay. Representative individual drug-naive human samples (diseased or non-diseased) from the population are tested during the assay validation to set screening and confirmatory cut points (as well as neutralizing cut point if any). In early phase studies, individual samples with the disease of interest may not be readily available to determine the cut points. Instead, healthy subjects are typically used. When targeted diseased subjects become available as the clinical program progresses to later clinical stages, it is necessary to use diseased subjects to re-establish the cut points if the previously determined cut points appear to be inadequate. Because of the potential risk of the biotherapeutics, it is desirable to have more false positives than false negatives. For clinical sample testing, FDA (2009) recommends a 5% false positive rate for the screening assay. A false positive rate of 1% or 0.1% is typically recommended for confirmatory assays (Shankar et al. (2008)). Neutralizing antibody assays use similar false positive rates (Gupta et al. (2011)). For preclinical studies, 1% or 0.1% false positive rate may be used (USP<1106>) for screening assays and confirmatory assays may be skipped. Because of the importance of cut points for ADA assay, a whole chapter (Chapter 3) is devoted to this topic.

2.2.1.2 Sensitivity

For ADA assays, due to the lack of reference standards, surrogate monoclonal and polyclonal ADAs are often used as positive control samples and also for calibration purposes. However, surrogate ADAs cannot truly represent human ADAs. Despite this limitation, surrogate ADAs are commonly used to determine assay sensitivity which is a regulatory expectation. According to FDA guidance (FDA (2009)), ADA assay sensitivity "represents the lowest concentration at which the antibody preparation consistently produces either a positive result or a readout equal to the cut point determined for that particular assay." For clinical studies, it is desirable to achieve a sensitivity of about 250–500 ng/mL .

To obtain dilution curves (standard curves), positive control samples with known high concentration are serially diluted until signals below the screening cut point. At least six curves are to be prepared by at least two analysts with each analyst conducting multiple runs. Positive controls should be prepared in pooled matrix in stead of individual samples matrices to remove the effect of biological variability. Negative controls should also be included. For biotherapeutics, dilution curves are often nonlinear. It is recommended to fit dilution curve data by appropriate nonlinear regression models in order to interpolate the concentration corresponding to the screening cut point. 95% consistency (confidence) is usually preferred because it guarantees that only 5% of time, the ADA with concentration at reported sensitivity will be misclassified as negative by the assay. To obtain the assay sensitivity, each dilution curve is interpolated to give rise to an ADA concentration corresponding to the screening cut point. The mean and standard deviation (SD) of the interpolated antibody concentrations from these dilution curves are used to calculate the reported assay sensitivity, i.e., $mean + t_{0.95,df} * SD$, where $t_{0.95,df}$ is the critical value covering 95% probability of the t-distribution (or 95% percentile) with degree-of-freedom being one less than the total number of dilution curves. The procedure is illustrated in Figure 2.2.

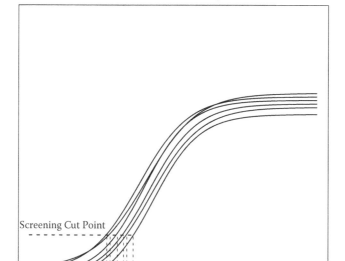

Dilution Curves from Multiple Runs

FIGURE 2.2
Illustration of a nonlinear dilution curve and interpolation.

The basic calibration curve is a four-parameter logistic model which has the following form:

$$y_j = d + (a - d)/(1 + (x_j/c)^b) + \epsilon_j \tag{2.1}$$

where y_j is the jth observed response at concentration x_j and b is the slope parameter. When $b > 0$, the concentration-response relationship is decreasing and vice versa for $b < 0$. a and d are the asymptotes as the concentration goes to zero and infinity, respectively. c is the inflection point around which the mean calibration curve is symmetric; it is the concentration corresponding to halfway between a and d (sometimes called EC50 in dose-response modelling)). There are some variations of the mathematical forms of logistic models, making the interpretation of the models rather confusing. Ritz (2010) gave a comprehensive review of dose-response models which include the four-parameter logistic model and made clarifications for the naming conventions. The aforementioned model (2.1) is better called log-logistic model. In contrast, the logistic model widely seen in literature has a slightly different form:

$$y_j = d + (a - d)/(1 + \exp\{b(x_j - c)\}) + \epsilon_j \tag{2.2}$$

This model (2.2) differs from model (2.1) in that x_j is the (natural) log-transformed concentration. In this case, the parameter c is in fact the log of EC50. Many software packages such as Prism require that the concentration is on log scale. However, when the concentration is exactly 0, a small positive number needs to be added to make the log transformation possible. Otherwise, the two models are essentially the same. However, inference results should be interpreted differently if one uses model (2.2) while treating x as on the original concentration.

The four-parameter logistic model may not be adequate due to asymmetry of actual dilution curve and a more general five-parameter logistic model may better characterize the concentration-response relationship of non-competitive assays. The five-parameter (log-)logistic model has the following form:

$$y_j = d + (a - d)/(1 + (x_j/c)^b)^g + \epsilon_j \tag{2.3}$$

This model allows for an asymmetric concentration-response relationship by adding an additional parameter g, which effectively allows the mean response function to approach the minimal or maximal response at different rates (Findlay and Dillard (2007)). In both of these models, ϵ_j is the intra-assay error term.

Nonlinear dilution curves may have nonconstant variance, meaning that as the ADA concentration increases, the variability of signals also increases. One way to correct for this is to take the log transformation for the signal or the more general Box–Cox transformation.[1] Alternatively, statistical techniques applicable to regression models can be utilized here for nonlinear calibration curves. The issue of variance heterogeneity does not affect the estimation of

---

[1]See Chapter 3 for an introduction to Box–Cox transformation.

regression parameters but does affect the variance of these estimators. Consequently, the estimated sensitivity will be affected. To correct for the variance heterogeneity, the method of weighted least square estimation is often used. The weighting scheme is well studied in the literature; see, for example, Davidian and Giltinan (1995). Consider the simple four-parameter (log)-logistic model of the following form:

$$y_{ij} = d_i + \frac{a_i - d_i}{1 + (x_{ij}/c_i)^{b_i}} + \epsilon_{ij} \tag{2.4}$$

where i refers to the ith curve and j stands for the jth concentration, ϵ_{ij} is the error term with mean 0 and unknown variance σ^2. In order to account for the nonconstant variance, O'Connell et al. (1993) considered a specific type of weighting function which works well empirically for immunoassays. Mathematically, they considered the following regression model:

$$y_{ij} = f(x_{ij}, \beta) + g[f(x_{ij}, \beta)]\epsilon_{ij} \tag{2.5}$$

where $f(x_{ij}, \beta)$ is the mean response curve such as the four-parameter logistic curve defined above with unknown parameter β, a vector representing all the unknown parameters for the curve. $g[f(x_{ij}, \beta)] = (f(x_{ij}, \beta))^\theta$ is a power function of the mean response at given a concentration, with unknown parameter θ to be estimated along with the variance parameter. Parameter estimation of a nonlinear regression curve with nonconstant variance is not trivial. Unlike the linear regression model, there is no closed-form solution and iteration is often needed to obtain parameter estimation.

While the method described by O'Connell et al. (1993) can stabilize the variance by using a common θ across different runs, it is possible that some of the individual curves cannot be fitted successfully. It is generally not recommended to exclude runs which fail the curve fitting due to significant loss of information. A better way to overcome this difficulty is to use nonlinear random effect model:

$$y_{ij} = d_i + \frac{a_i - d_i}{1 + (x_{ij}/c_i)^{b_i}} + \epsilon_{ij} \tag{2.6}$$

where the parameters a_i, b_i, c_i, d_i are assumed to be random and follow a multivariate normal distribution $N(\mu, \Sigma)$ where $\mu = (a, b, c, d)$ is the mean vector and Σ is a diagonal covariance matrix in its simplest form. After the model is fitted, the sensitivity can be calculated as the interpolation of the lower 95% confidence limit of the mean calibration curve from the cut point. The variance of the interpolated concentration can be calculated accordingly. The SAS procedure PROC MIXED and the R packages `nlme` or `lme4` can fit nonlinear random effect model. Alternatively, Bayesian analysis can be used for inference via simulation method such as Markov chain Monte Carlo (MCMC).

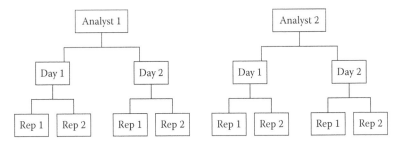

FIGURE 2.3
Illustration of a simple precision design of experiment.

2.2.1.3 Drug Tolerance

Drug tolerance or drug interference is part of the selectivity/interference study. Selectivity is the ability of an assay to measure the analyte of interest in the presence of interfering factors such as the drug itself, concomitant medications, rheumatoid factor.

Because the study drug itself can bind to the ADAs, it can compete with the labeled drug during sample testing. Therefore, it is usually the main interferant in an ADA assay. The drug tolerance is defined as the highest concentration of drug that positive samples remain detectable. Investigation of the drug tolerance is often a regulatory expectation. During assay validation studies, the low ADA quality control samples are pre-incubated with serial dilutions of the drug and then tested in the assay. The lowest concentration of drug that classifies the quality control sample as positive is the drug tolerance. Note that the drug tolerance, like sensitivity, is highly dependent on the positive control samples used. Several articles discuss drug interference including Zhong et al. (2010) and Barbosa et al. (2012).

2.2.1.4 Precision

The precision of an assay describes the closeness of individual measurements of an analyte when the procedure is applied repeatedly to multiple aliquots of a single homogeneous sample. Precision demonstrates the assay reproducibility and is thus critical to the assessment of immunogenicity. Precision is often evaluated using positive control (low positive and high positive) samples. Samples are tested in multiple validation runs to evaluate both intra-assay (repeatability) and inter-assay (intermediate precision) variability of assay responses. Inter-assay variability reflects the variability that is unavoidable under routine laboratory sample testing due to various laboratory conditions such as analyst, instrument, and plate. Consequently, the inter-assay variability includes several components such as analyst-to-analyst variability, day-to-day variability, etc.

Data from replicates of positive control samples are often used to report precision. Random effect (variance component) ANOVA model is useful to estimate various variance components. Figure 2.3 illustrates a simple nested design for a precision study. In this study design, there are two analysts; two days are nested within each analyst. Two replicates are performed on each day by each analyst. The ANOVA model is denoted as

$$y_{ijk} = \mu + \alpha_i + \beta_{j(i)} + \epsilon_{ijk} \tag{2.7}$$

where α_i and $\beta_{j(i)}$ denote the random effect of the ith analyst on the jth day. α_i, $\beta_{j(i)}$ and ϵ_{ijk} are assumed to be independently normal random variables with mean 0 and variances σ_α^2, σ_β^2 and σ_ϵ^2, respectively. The variances σ_α^2, σ_β^2 and σ_ϵ^2 refer to the analyst-to-analyst, day-to-day, and intra-assay variabilities, respectively. The variance component estimates can be derived from the following ANOVA table:

TABLE 2.1
ANOVA table for nested model

Source	SS	DF	MS	EMS
Analyst	SS_A	$I-1$	MS_A	$\sigma_\epsilon^2 + K\sigma_\beta^2 + JK\sigma_\alpha^2$
Day(Analyst)	SS_B	$I(J-1)$	MS_B	$\sigma_\epsilon^2 + K\sigma_\beta^2$
Error	SS_E	$IJ(K-1)$	MS_E	σ_ϵ^2
Total	$SSTO$	$IJK-1$		

where $MS_A = SS_A/(I-1)$, $MS_B = SS_B/(I(J-1))$ and $MS_E = SS_E/(IJ(K-1)))$.

The total sum of square $SSTO$ breaks down as follows:

$$\sum_{i=1}^{I}\sum_{j=1}^{J}\sum_{k=1}^{K}(y_{ijk} - \bar{y})^2 = JK\sum_{i=1}^{I}(\bar{y}_i - \bar{y})^2 +$$

$$K\sum_{i=1}^{I}\sum_{j=1}^{J}(\bar{y}_{ij} - \bar{y}_i)^2 + \sum_{i=1}^{I}\sum_{j=1}^{J}\sum_{k=1}^{K}(y_{ijk} - \bar{y}_{ij})^2 \tag{2.8}$$

where $\bar{y}_{ij} = \sum_{k=1}^{K}y_{ijk}/K$, $\bar{y}_i = \sum_{j=1}^{J}\sum_{k=1}^{K}y_{ijk}/JK$, and $\bar{y} = \sum_{i=1}^{I}\sum_{j=1}^{J}\sum_{k=1}^{K}y_{ijk}/IJK$. The notations used in Table 2.1, SS_A, SS_B and SS_E refer to the three terms on the right side of equation (2.8) in that order. The mean sum-of-squares MS_A, MS_B and MS_E intend to measure the variation due to analyst, day within analyst and the error term, respectively. However, because data for the same analyst are actually correlated, what they measure has the expectation in those terms as shown in the last column of Table 2.1. By equating the mean square in the second to last column to the expected mean square in the last column in Table 2.1, the variance components can be estimated by solving the equations, resulting in the following parameter estimates:

$$
\begin{aligned}
\hat{\sigma}_{\epsilon}^2 &= MS_E \\
\hat{\sigma}_{\beta}^2 &= (MS_B - MS_E)/K \\
\hat{\sigma}_{\alpha}^2 &= (MS_A - MS_B)/JK
\end{aligned}
$$

This estimation method is essentially the method of moment.

Computer software packages often use the restricted maximum likelihood estimation (REML) for parameter estimations. The REML method and the above-mentioned method of moment lead to the same result when the data/design structure is balanced. The R functions *lme* in R package `nlme` or the *lmer* function in R package `lme4` can be used. The SAS procedures PROC GLM and PROC MIXED can be used for nested random effect ANOVA model.

2.2.1.5 Robustness

Assay robustness is an indication of the assay's reliability during normal day-to-day usage. Assay robustness is to assess the capacity of the assay to remain within specification ranges when small but deliberate changes, that would be expected during real sample testing in the laboratory, are made deliberately. The typical variables chosen for robustness testing include incubation times, reagent lot, reagent concentration, and sample freeze-thaw cycles, to name a few. Assay robustness is often explored after assay optimization or during assay validation. However, it is advised that robustness testing be initiated early in assay development and validation. This is because if the assay does not meet the criteria for robustness early enough in development, there may not be enough time to re-optimize the assay before formal pre-study validation. In effect, this delay could increase overall turnaround time and development cost.

2.2.1.6 Ruggedness/Reproducibility

Ruggedness/reproducibility testing is an assessment of agreement of data from samples tested at different laboratories. This often occurs in assay transfer. When an the assay is transferred to a different laboratory, a comparability study comparing data generated in the original lab to those in the new lab is required. In section 2.4, statistical method regarding data agreement is introduced.

2.2.2 Life-Cycle Approach

After pre-study validation, the assay is ready for in-study sample testing. During this stage, the validated assay needs to be continually monitored for its performance. Generally, validation of an assay does not end until the method is no longer in use or is replaced by another assay. During the use of the assay, various conditions may change, e.g., reagents due to vendor changes, equipment, analysts. Depending on the changes, the assay may either need to be partially or fully revalidated. Under circumstances where partial revalidation is sufficient, only critical assay performance parameters will be re-assessed.

2.3 Design of Experiment

DOE has been used in various fields, starting in agriculture in early twentieth century and later applied to industry product and process optimization. The application of DOE to assay development has been increasingly popular (see, Ray et al. (2009), Joelsson et al. (2008), Chen et al. (2012)). Civoli et al. (2012) gave a nice review of NAb assay development and optimization using DOE method. In assay optimization, scientists who are unaware of DOE often try to optimize the assay by varying the level of assay variables (in statistics, they are called factors) one at a time. This process can, however, be very time and resource consuming. The traditional one factor at a time (OFAT) technique may take many steps to reach a target endpoint without realizing that factors are affecting the results in an interactive nature, leading to incomplete understanding of the behavior of the assay. Using DOE, the assay conditions can be varied simultaneously. Therefore, DOE is an effective way for assay optimization. In this section, several popular designs are introduced briefly with applications to immunogenicity assay. Several books (Haaland (1989), Montgomery (2008)) are devoted to the topic of DOE. Interested readers are encouraged to consult these books for more details. Before introducing DOE, it is helpful to introduce some terminology particular to DOEs.

- Factor: any assay variable such as analyst, instrument, incubation time, reagent concentration, minimum required dilution.

- Factor Level: a particular value for a factor. Factors such as instrument can only take a few nominal values (e.g., instrument 1 and 2), while factors such as incubation time can theoretically take any positive real numbers.

- Treatment: a particular combination of factor levels.

- Response: the endpoint of interest in an experiment. There may be several responses of interest in an experiment.

- Factor Effect: the change in response caused by changes in levels of a factor.

- Interaction Effect: the change in response of one factor is not the same at different levels of another factor. Interaction effect is the joint contribution of several factors on the response.

- Experimental Unit: an experimental unit is the smallest division of the experimental material such that any two experimental units can receive different treatments.

Key to utilizing DOE correctly and effectively is to understand the basic principles of experimental designs, namely, randomization, replication and blocking.

- *Randomization.* Randomization is the cornerstone of all the statistical methods. It is the assignment of treatments to the experimental units so that each treatment has equal chance of being assigned to the experimental unit. Randomization is often achieved using computer software or some specific randomization scheme. The purpose of randomization is to eliminate (or average out) the effect of other sources of variation, which are not under consideration or not controllable. Unfortunately, complete randomization is sometimes not possible due to some restrictions. For example, it is difficult to vary temperature within a single assay plate.

- *Replication.* Replication is an independent repetition (or run) of the experiment for all the treatments. In contrast, duplication refers to the multiple measurements for the same run. Replication allows the investigator to accurately estimate the experimental error, on which the statistical inference of factor effects are based, such as testing significance or constructing confidence intervals. By increasing the number of replications, the experimental error will be reduced and consequently the factor effect estimation will be more precise. This can be best illustrated by the following example. Given sample mean $\bar{y}$ in the simple independently and identically distribution (IID) normal case where $y_1, \cdots, y_n \sim N(\mu, \sigma^2)$, increasing the number of sample n will reduce the standard error $\sigma/\sqrt{n}$ of the sample mean.

- *Blocking.* Some nuisance factors which are not of main interest may have an effect on the statistical inference. Randomization and replication may not be enough to eliminate the effect of these nuisance factors. Blocking is an effective way to reduce the impact of these nuisance factors. Blocking means to group the experimental units in relatively homogeneous groups. Randomization is then applied to each of these groups. The main purpose of blocking is to increase the efficiency of an experimental design by decreasing the experimental error.

There are many well-known designs. The choice of these designs depends on the study purpose and circumstances. In the following, many of the named designs are introduced.

2.3.1 Fractional Factorial Design

Fractional factorial design is the most common design used to investigate effects of factors and their interactions. It is particularly useful when the number of experimental factors being considered makes it unfeasible to use traditional factorial design (or full factorial design) due to efficiency and cost issues. For instance, in traditional full factorial design, each factor takes two levels (low level and high level). For two factors with two levels for each factor, four runs are needed to explore every combination of the two factors. For three factors, eight runs are needed. In general, for k factors, 2^k runs are needed. The number of runs increases exponentially for full factorials with only two levels as the number of factors increases. This method quickly becomes unfeasible. Fractional factorial design offers a solution to this issue. The fractional factorial design uses a fraction of the number of runs of full factorial design by sacrificing the high order interactions terms. A technical description of how fractional factorial designs are constructed is beyond the scope of this introduction. To illustrate the idea, consider the following simple example: a full five-factor, two-level design to study the effects of Temperature, Capture incubation time, Detection incubation time and two other plate factors[2] in an ELISA bridging assay for immunogenicity testing. A full factorial design would require $2^5 = 32$ runs. While this design, to be performed by a single analyst, may be reasonably affordable, it may be unnecessary in practice. In a half-fraction factorial design, only 16 (2^{5-1}) runs are needed. This effectively saves resources and turnaround times. This hypothetical 16-run design is depicted in Table 2.2 and can be constructed easily using software such as JMP. The design displayed below should be interpreted as follows. Each column contains +1's or -1's to indicate the setting of each factor (high or low level). For example, in the first run of the experiment, Capture incubation time, Detection incubation time and Var 5 all take their high level values; while both Temperature and Var 4 take their low level values. Note that the first column Order, list the randomized order of the runs, which is typically provided by DOE software.

For full factorial design, all the effects including main effects, two-factor interaction effects, and high-order interaction effects can be estimated. However, in practice, it is often the case that the high-order interaction effects can be assumed to be negligible. With only 5 main factor effects and up to 10 two-factor interaction effects to be estimated, an experiment with 16 runs would be able to estimate these effects. The one-half fractional factorial design is fit for this purpose, effectively reducing the resources by a half when compared with a full factorial design. However, it is probably not good in this example to further reduce the 16-run design to 8-run design, or one-quarter fractional factorial design. The reason is that some factor effect will be confounded or aliased with other factor effects, making a clear separation of all low-order factor effects impossible. By confounding or aliasing, factor (main or interaction)

---

[2]By plate factors, factor levels are the same for a whole plate.

TABLE 2.2

Fractional factorial design for five factors

Order	Temp	Capture time	Detection time	Var 4	Var 5
1	-1	1	1	-1	1
2	1	-1	-1	-1	-1
3	-1	-1	1	1	1
4	1	1	1	-1	-1
5	1	1	-1	1	-1
6	-1	-1	-1	1	-1
7	-1	1	1	1	-1
8	-1	-1	-1	-1	1
9	1	1	1	1	1
10	1	-1	1	-1	1
11	-1	1	-1	1	1
12	1	1	-1	-1	1
13	-1	-1	1	-1	-1
14	1	-1	1	1	-1
15	-1	1	-1	-1	-1
16	1	-1	-1	1	1

effects can only be estimated together and are thus unable to be separated out from one another. The one-quarter fractional factorial design is still useful in some cases where the two-factor effects are not important such as in screening design to be introduced later. When selecting fractional factorial design, it is important to understand the aliasing in the design. This is also called design resolution. Resolution III, IV, and V are the most important ones.

- Resolution III design: designs in which no main effect is aliased with any other main effects, but main effects are aliased with two-factor interactions and some two-factor interactions may be aliased with one another.

- Resolution IV design: designs in which no main effect is aliased with any other main effect or with any two-factor interaction, but two-factor interactions are aliased with each other.

- Resolution V design: designs in which no main effect or two-factor interaction is aliased with any other main effects or two-factor interactions, although two factor interactions are aliased with three-factor interactions.

Many DOE softwares such as JMP and Design-Expert provide design choices with different resolutions. For example, Figure 2.4 is from Design-Expert. For a given number of factors (column), the table gives all the possible fractional factorial designs with different resolutions. For example, when the number of factors is 6, a resolution III design requires 8 runs and is denoted as 2^{6-3}_{III}, where the subscript denotes the resolution.

	2	3	4	5	6	7	8	9	10	11	12
4	2^2	2^{3-1}_{III}									
8		2^3	2^{4-1}_{IV}	2^{5-2}_{III}	2^{6-3}_{III}	2^{7-4}_{III}					
16			2^4	2^{5-1}_{V}	2^{6-2}_{IV}	2^{7-3}_{IV}	2^{8-4}_{IV}	2^{9-5}_{III}	2^{10-6}_{III}	2^{11-7}_{III}	2^{12-8}_{III}
32				2^5	2^{6-1}_{VI}	2^{7-2}_{IV}	2^{8-3}_{IV}	2^{9-4}_{IV}	2^{10-5}_{IV}	2^{11-6}_{IV}	2^{12-7}_{IV}
64					2^6	2^{7-1}_{VII}	2^{8-2}_{V}	2^{9-3}_{IV}	2^{10-4}_{IV}	2^{11-5}_{IV}	2^{12-6}_{IV}
128						2^7	2^{8-1}_{VIII}	2^{9-2}_{VI}	2^{10-3}_{V}	2^{11-4}_{V}	2^{12-5}_{IV}
256							2^8	2^{9-1}_{IX}	2^{10-2}_{VI}	2^{11-3}_{VI}	2^{12-4}_{VI}
512								2^9	2^{10-1}_{X}	2^{11-2}_{VII}	2^{12-3}_{VI}

FIGURE 2.4

Factorial design resolution table.

The fractional factorial design is very useful as a screening design when there is limited knowledge of an assay (or a system in general) initially, say, at the beginning of assay development. To begin, factors are brainstormed and those suspected to have effects on the response of interest are under consideration, but only a few are believed to have significant effects. Screening design is an efficient way to separate those few important factors from the many.

Another popular design is called Plackett–Burman design. Unlike the fractional factorial design, in which the number of runs is always a power of 2, the number of runs for Plackett–Burman design is a multiple of 4, making it flexible if the experimenter can only afford 12, 20, 28, ... , runs. The Plackett–Burman design is a resolution III design, which means that all the two-factor interactions are confounded with some of the main-factor effects. It is then best suited for screening purposes where it is believed that two-factor interaction effects are negligible. Plackett–Burman designs allow one to check the main factors effect with the least number of runs. In the assay robustness study, if the interaction effects are believed to be negligible, the Plackett–Burman design is a time and resource efficient design to use. For assay robustness, Vander Heyden et al. (2001) gave a comprehensive review of the statistical designs with emphasis on Plackett–Burman design and related data analysis for small molecule analytical methods. This approach is also applicable to immunogenicity assay robustness study.

2.3.2 Response Surface Design

To optimize a process or an assay, statistical design is useful to find the best combination of factor levels or a region where the process or assay satisfactorily achieves its response target. Due to the complexity of the interplay of many factors, the mechanistic model describing the response as a function of the factors is often not available or difficult to obtain. Mathematically, the mechanistic model can be described as:

$$y = f(x_1, x_2, \ldots, x_k) + \epsilon \tag{2.9}$$

The functional form may not be known. However, low-order polynomials such as first-order and second-order polynomials are found to be good approximations. Using statistical designs and regression techniques applied to the collected data, an empirical model can be built for the process or assay. The problem of optimizing a process is often conquered sequentially. First, screening designs with many unknown factors are performed to extract the possible important factors and interactions. Second, a response surface design is applied using the extracted factors to build a response surface for optimization; see Figure 2.5 for a typical response surface with two factors. The entire se-

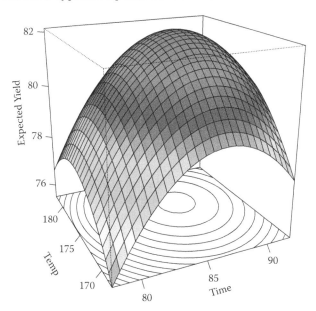

FIGURE 2.5
A typical response surface graph with the maximal response in the center of the region.

quence of experiments to build a satisfactory response surface is not straight-forward. This is an area that scientists and statisticians can work together to make meaningful progress. From a design perspective, the process of building a response surface is much like hiking to the summit of a mountain. In the first step, the correct direction toward the summit must be identified. Once the direction is pinpointed, further movement along the direction should be continued until the surrounding of the summit is nearby. Finally, more sophisticated strategy may be applied to reach the summit confidently. The theory and practice of response surface design is rather rich and several books are devoted to this topic. The reader can refer to Myers et al. (2009) for more details.

Sometimes the region of interest may not contain the optimum. It is thus important to differentiate different shapes of response surface mathematically as well as visually. Figure 2.6 shows the different shapes of response surface from two factors. In the first graph (upper left), the maximum is reached. In the second graph (upper right), neither a minimum nor maximum exists, which indicates a search for the optimum in a different region is required. In the last graph (bottom), the optimum is reached with respect with the second factor only, because the response is linear with respect to the first factor.

Two commonly used response surface designs are central composite design (CCD) and Box–Behnken design (Box and Behnken (1960)). These two designs have nice properties as described below and should be utilized in practice whenever possible. The CCD design is a natural extension of the 2-level full factorial design by adding center runs as well as extended axial runs. Figure 2.7 (left) shows a CCD design for two factors. There are five levels for each factor, so that in addition to the main effect and interaction effects, it is possible to estimate quadratic terms. The distance between the center point and each axial point is $\sqrt{2}$ or 1.414. Each non-central point has the same distance to the center. It has the property of equal variance of predicted response at these external design points, which is known as *rotatability*. The CCD design is said to be *on face* if the axial values are shrunk to -1 and 1. The face-centered CCD only requires three factor levels (for each factor) at the potential cost of losing some estimation precision. One advantage of rotatable CCD is that when blocking is necessary, the block effect does not affect the other factor effects.

Another popular response surface design is the Box–Behnken design. The Box–Behnken design is a 3-level design with design points at the centers of the edges instead of the corners. The Box–Behnken design is either rotatable or nearly rotatable. It differs from CCD in that the design points are not at the corners of the design space and is thus most appropriate when the combination of factor levels at the extreme is not feasible.

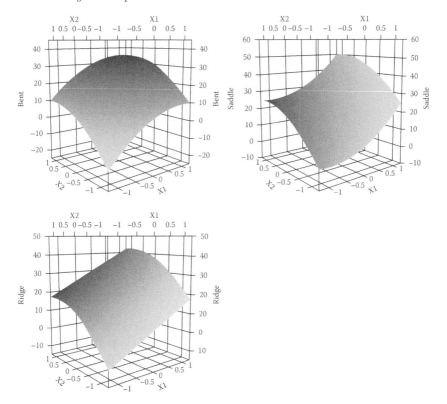

FIGURE 2.6

Different shape of response surface. In the upper left graph, the maximum is reached. In the upper right graph, neither maximum nor minimum is in the region. In the bottom graph, the maximum is with respect to the second factor but not the first factor.

2.3.3 Split-Plot Design

For plate-based assays, it is common to have some factors that can be changed easily within the plate, such as reagent concentration, while other factors such as temperature are relatively hard to change and better kept the same for the whole plate. This restricts randomization of some factors with respect to

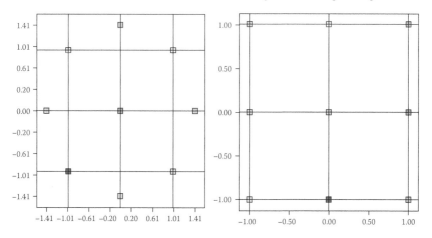

FIGURE 2.7
Central composite design for two factors. Left: Regular CCD; Right: Face-centered CCD.

plates. Split-plot designs can accommodate such restrictions. Many experiments previously thought to be completely randomized experiments actually exhibit split-plot structure. A split-plot design is a blocked design where the blocks serve as experimental units for the hard-to-change factors. Therefore, there are two levels of experimental units. The blocks are called whole plot, while the experimental units within blocks are called subplots. Box et al. (2005) described an example of split-plot design to demonstrate the importance of recognizing correct design structure and applying an appropriate method for data analysis. In their example, the experiment was designed to study the corrosion resistance of steel bars treated with four `Coatings`, C_1, C_2, C_3, and C_4, at three furnace `Temperatures`, $360°C, 370°C$ and $380°C$. The positions of the coated steel bars in the furnace were randomized within each temperature setting. However, because the furnace temperature was difficult to change, the temperature settings were run in a systematic order rather than randomly. Table 2.3 shows the results from a split-plot experiment where the whole plot is replicated twice, resulting in six whole plots and four subplots within each whole plot.

The data structure of split-plot experiments such as in Table 2.3 is similar to that from a completely randomized design. However, the data analyses due to the two different designs are different. Table 2.4 provides p-values for testing the significance of the effects in the corrosion-resistance example. At the significance level of 0.05, the appropriate analysis for the split-plot design shows that `coating` and the interaction between `Temperature` and `Coating` are significant. However, if the experimenter analyzes the data as a completely randomized design, the results are reversed. As shown in Table 2.4, the effect

TABLE 2.3

Example of split-plot design

Furnace Run(Whole Plot)	Temperature	Coating			
1	360	67	73	83	89
2	370	65	91	87	86
3	380	155	127	147	212
4	380	108	100	90	153
5	370	140	142	121	150
6	360	33	8	46	54

of Temperature is statistically significant while the other two effects are not significant.

TABLE 2.4

P-values for corrosion-resistance example

Effect	Split-plot design	CRD[a]
Temperature(A)	0.209	0.003
Coating(B)	0.002	0.386
Temperature× Coating (A× B)	0.024	0.852

[a] CRD: Completely randomized design.

In the analysis of split-plot designs, the whole plots and subplots form two different types of experiment units. As a result, there are two different error terms: whole plot error and subplot error. To test the effect significance, the whole plot effects are compared to the whole plot error and to test the significance of all the other effects, they are compared to the subplot error. The statistical model for a split-plot design can be written as

$$y_{ijk} = \mu + \alpha_i + \delta_{ik} + \beta_j + (\alpha\beta)_{ij} + \epsilon_{ijk} \tag{2.10}$$

where μ is the overall mean, α_i is the whole plot factor (e.g., Temperature in the corrosion resistance example), δ_{ik} is the whole plot error (representing the random effect for the kth whole plot at the ith level of A), β_j is the subplot factor (e.g., Coating), $(\alpha\beta)_{ij}$ is the interaction (e.g., Temperature× Coating) effect, and ϵ_{ijk} is the subplot error. δ_{ik} is assumed to be normally distributed with mean 0 and variance σ_{WP}^2; ϵ_{ijk} is assumed to be independent of δ_{ik} and normally distributed with mean 0 and variance σ_{SP}^2. The ANOVA table for the split-plot analysis is as follows:

The ANOVA table of split-plot design is different from that of a completely randomized design in that the break-up of the total sum-of-squares as well as the degrees-of-freedom are different. Consequently, the expected mean square

TABLE 2.5

ANOVA table for a split-plot design

Source	SS	DF	Expected MS (EMS)
Factor A	SS_A	$I-1$	$\sigma_{SP}^2 + J\sigma_{WP}^2 + JK\sum_{i=1}^{I}\alpha_i^2/(I-1)$
Whole Plot Error	$SS(A)$	$I(K-1)$	$\sigma_{SP}^2 + J\sigma_{WP}^2$
Factor B	SS_B	$J-1$	$\sigma_{SP}^2 + IK\sum_{j=1}^{J}\beta_j^2/(J-1)$
Interaction AB	SS_{AB}	$(I-1)(J-1)$	$\sigma_{SP}^2 + \frac{K\sum_{i=1}^{I}\sum_{j=1}^{J}(\alpha\beta)_{ij}^2}{(I-1)(J-1)}$
Subplot Error	SSE	$I(J-1)(K-1)$	σ_{SP}^2
Total	SST	$IJK-1$	

of each factor effect is also different. To test the significance of the effect of factor A, the whole plot error should be used in the denominator of the F-test. When there are more than two factors, the ANOVA table is rather complicated. For example, when there are three whole plot factors A, B, and C and two subplot factors D, and E, the interaction between D and E should be compared to whole plot error, because this interaction effect is aliased with the whole plot effects, assuming all the high-order interaction effects are negligible; for details, see section 14.5 of Montgomery (2008).

JMP custom design can be used to make a split-plot design. Figure 2.8 illustrates how to make split-plot design for the corrosion resistance example. By default, one replication ($K = 2$) is performed in JMP, leading to six whole plots in the corrosion resistance example.

When the number of factors gets larger, fractional factorial design or Plackett–Burman is often used to reduce the total number of runs. Incorporation of fractional factorial design or Plackett–Burman design into a split-plot structure is possible, but rather complicated. This is an active area of research currently. Similarly, the split-plot structure also appears in response surface design.

2.3.4   Design Optimality

Often, it is not uncommon that the aforementioned designs cannot be directly applied simply because some of the factor combinations are not feasible or scientists have other considerations. One reasonable compromise in such situations is to choose factor combinations from the available ranges such that certain optimal criterion is met. Among the designs with most common criterion are the so-called D-optimal designs. The D-optimal design is a useful compromise when experimental constraints prevent adoption of the standard designs discussed above. The D-optimal criterion is to maximize the determinant of information matrix such that the overall variance of the parameter estimations is minimized. The D-optimal design is appropriate for screening design, where the goal is to test significance of factor effects.

For response surface design problems, the main objective of the design

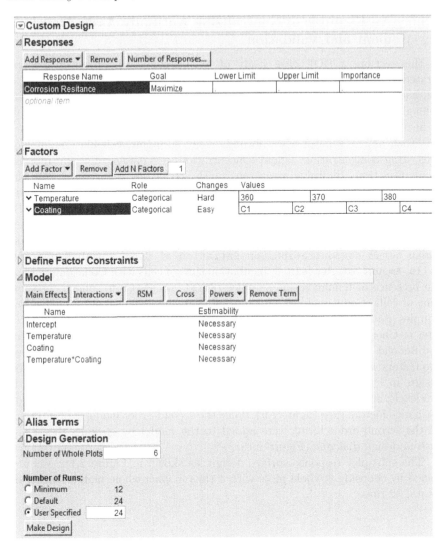

FIGURE 2.8
Split-plot design in JMP.

and analysis is to predict and obtain the most precise response. For this purpose, the I-optimal criterion is more appropriate than the D-optimal criterion. The I-optimal criterion minimizes the average variance of prediction over the experimental design region. The I-optimal design has the lowest prediction variance near the center of the design space where the optimal response is more likely located.

2.3.5 An Example of Neutralizing Antibody Assay Development and Validation

In this section, a DOE case study of NAb assay development is demonstrated based on the example by Chen et al. (2012). In their example, a cell-based bioassay was developed for the detection of NAbs against a monoclonal antibody drug under development. An indirect assay format (Civoli et al. (2012)) was adopted. During the assay development stage, many factors such as the type of assay format, assay endpoint, cell line, number of cells, drug concentration, ligand concentration, percentage of serum matrix, incubation time, desirable assay sensitivity need to be determined. Subject matter knowledge along with past experience can be utilized to determine some of the factors such as cell line and assay format. In Chen et al. (2012), an H2122 human non-small cell lung cancer cell line was chosen and it is decided to directly apply response surface design with the following six factors: `Human serum concentration`, `Concentration of Conatumumab`, `Number of cells`, `Amount of Protein G`, incubation time of cells with Conatumumab in the presence of human serum samples (`First incubation`), and incubation time of cells, Conatumumab and protein G in the presence of human serum samples (`Second incubation`). For the detailed assay development procedure, refer to Chen et al. (2012). Because some factors, such as `First incubation` and `Second incubation` times, are difficult to vary within a plate and these two factors were evaluated plate by plate, Chen et al. (2012) chose a split-plot design. In JMP custom design, the factors were set to continuous factors with two levels; and `First incubation` and `Second incubation` were set to hard-to-change factors (See Figure 2.9). Since the second-order model is of interest, all the second-order terms were added to the model by clicking "RSM" in custom design dialogue (Figure 2.10).

The split-plot response surface design, as shown in Figure 2.11, was obtained by choosing 8 whole plots with 4 runs in each whole plot, resulting in a total 32 runs.

2.4 Method Transfer

An assay developed and validated in one laboratory often needs to be transferred to another laboratory for various reasons, with the general aim to optimize resource utilization and improve overall efficiency. There is no guidance on controlling assay performance during immunogenicity assay transfer. However, comparing assay performance of original assay and transferred assay is necessary and successful assay transfer would increase the confidence. Therefore, assay transfers need to be carefully planned and executed.

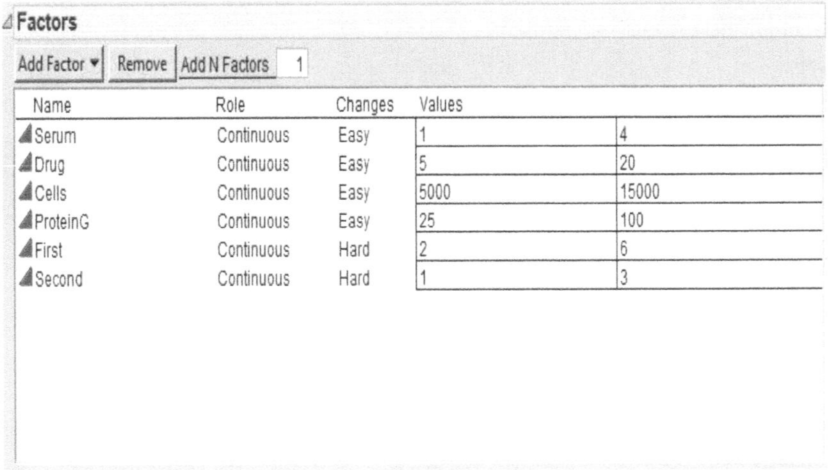

⊿ **Factors**					
Add Factor ▾ Remove Add N Factors 1					
Name	Role	Changes	Values		
⊿Serum	Continuous	Easy	1		4
⊿Drug	Continuous	Easy	5		20
⊿Cells	Continuous	Easy	5000		15000
⊿ProteinG	Continuous	Easy	25		100
⊿First	Continuous	Hard	2		6
⊿Second	Continuous	Hard	1		3

FIGURE 2.9
Factor setting in JMP custom design.

Tatarewicz et al. (2009) developed a three-step statistical approach to immunogenicity assay transfer. In the first step, the effect of key assay factors are studied and the mean equivalence of assay signals from individual donor samples of two labs are tested. To test for the equivalence of average assay signals from two labs, the two one-sided t-test (TOST) can be used. The TOST is different from the classical t-test in that the purpose of t-test is to test against the mean equality of two groups. In the classical two-sample (group) t-test, the hypothesis is formulated as follows:

$$H_0 : \mu_1 = \mu_2 \quad \text{v.s} \quad H_a : \mu_1 \neq \mu_2 \tag{2.11}$$

where μ_1 and μ_2 represent the mean of samples from the two independent groups, say lab 1 and lab 2. In the theory of hypothesis, the purpose of classical t-test is to support the alternative hypothesis, namely, to prove that there is a significant difference between the two group means, μ_1 and μ_2. Failure to reject the null hypothesis does not mean that the two group means are equal; rather, it indicates there is not enough evidence to disprove H_0. If the sample size increases, chances are that any small difference between μ_1 and μ_2 eventually will be detected by the t-test. On the other hand, to prove equivalence, the null and alternative hypotheses in (2.11) should be in other way around. Formally, in an equivalence test of two groups means, the hypothesis is:

$$H_0 : |\mu_1 - \mu_2| > \delta \quad \text{v.s} \quad H_a : |\mu_1 - \mu_2| \leq \delta$$

where δ is the equivalence bound for negligible difference of two group means, within which, the two group means can be deemed equivalent. Specification of δ should rely on subject matter expert knowledge. In testing for immunogenicity assay mean equivalence, $\delta = 0.223$ was used by Tatarewicz et al. (2009).

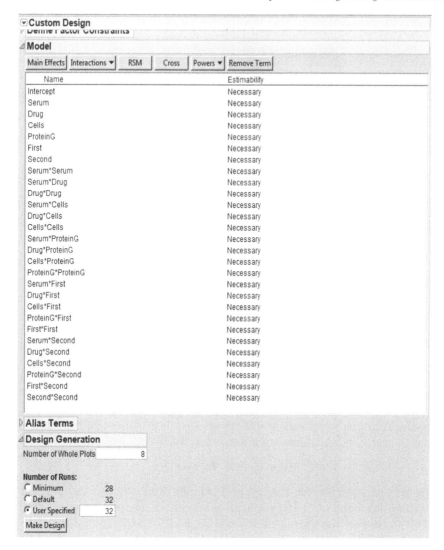

FIGURE 2.10
Response surface model specification in JMP custom design.

Note that the means mentioned here are all on the natural logarithm scale. The number 0.223 is borrowed from the equivalence criterion recommended for bioequivalence establishment (FDA (2001)).

As argued by Schuirmann (1987), the equivalence hypothesis is essentially

	Whole Plots	Serum	Drug	Cells	ProteinG	First	Second
1	1	2.5	5	15000	100	6	1
2	1	2.5	20	15000	25	6	1
3	1	1	5	5000	25	6	1
4	1	2.5	20	5000	100	6	1
5	2	4	5	5000	100	2	1
6	2	1	20	5000	25	2	1
7	2	1	5	10000	62.5	2	1
8	2	4	12.5	15000	25	2	1
9	3	4	12.5	10000	100	4	2
10	3	2.5	12.5	10000	62.5	4	2
11	3	2.5	5	15000	25	4	2
12	3	4	20	5000	25	4	2
13	4	2.5	12.5	10000	25	6	3
14	4	1	5	15000	100	6	3
15	4	4	20	5000	100	6	3
16	4	2.5	20	15000	62.5	6	3
17	5	4	20	5000	62.5	2	2
18	5	1	12.5	15000	25	2	2
19	5	2.5	12.5	15000	100	2	2
20	5	2.5	5	5000	25	2	2
21	6	4	5	5000	62.5	6	2
22	6	1	20	10000	62.5	6	2
23	6	4	12.5	15000	25	6	2
24	6	1	5	5000	100	6	2
25	7	4	5	10000	62.5	2	3
26	7	2.5	20	15000	25	2	3
27	7	1	12.5	5000	62.5	2	3
28	7	1	20	10000	100	2	3
29	8	4	20	15000	100	4	1
30	8	1	20	15000	100	4	1
31	8	4	5	15000	62.5	4	1
32	8	2.5	12.5	10000	62.5	4	1

FIGURE 2.11
Generation of response surface design table.

an interval hypothesis and can be decomposed into two sets of one-sided hypotheses:

$$H_{01} : \mu_1 - \mu_2 < -\delta \quad \text{v.s.} \quad H_{a1} : \mu_1 - \mu_2 \geq -\delta$$

and

$$H_{02} : \mu_1 - \mu_2 > \delta \quad \text{v.s.} \quad H_{a2} : \mu_1 - \mu_2 \leq \delta$$

If both H_{01} and H_{02} are rejected at the significance level α, then H_0 is also rejected at significance level α and equivalence is concluded. The classical one-sided t-test can be utilized for testing H_{01} and H_{02}, and thus the so-called two one-sided t-test or TOST. Operationally, it is equivalent to that

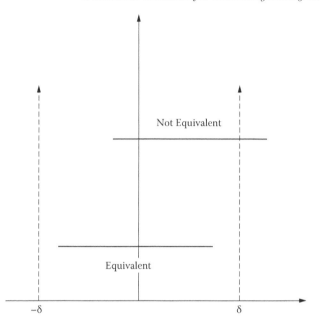

FIGURE 2.12
Illustration of equivalence test.

if the $(1 - 2\alpha)$ confidence interval is within $(-\delta, \delta)$, then H_0 is rejected, as illustrated in Figure 2.12. Berger and Hsu (1996) reviewed the theoretical framework of interaction union test (IUT) with equivalence test as a special case.

As pointed out by Zhong et al. (2008), the approach of equivalence testing is appropriate for comparing means between the source laboratory and the transfer laboratory. It is not enough for assays such as immunogenicity assay whose final purpose is to determine the positivity and titer of individual subjects. Therefore, some approach to establishing individual equivalence should be considered.

In the second step, Tatarewicz et al. (2009) proposed to assess assay agreement between source and transfer labs. In this evaluation, individual samples are assayed to determine whether data from the two labs are concordant. The Lin's coefficient of concordance correlation (CCC) was used by Tatarewicz et al. (2009). Before Lin's CCC was proposed, several methods such as the Pearson correlation coefficient, the paired t-test, least-squares regression, and intraclass correlation coefficient were used to evaluate agreement. As argued by Lin (1989), these methods do not take into account both the bias and variance of the data and thus can lead to misleading conclusion. For example, a very high Pearson correlation coefficient does not mean that the two group of data agree with each other. The paired data may fit tightly along a straight line other than the 45 line with intercept 0 and slope 1 on a plot. Figure 1-3 of Lin (1989) illustrated graphically the weaknesses of each method for assessing data agreement.

By taking the bias and variability into account simultaneously, Lin (1989) proposed to use a single index to assess data agreement. The rationale is as follows. Consider pairs of data $(Y_{i1}, Y_{i2}), i = 1, \ldots, n$ are independently from bivariate normal distribution with mean (μ_1, μ_2), variances (σ_1^2, σ_2^2) and correlation coefficient ρ. The degree of concordance between a pair of measurements (Y_1, Y_2) from two labs is defined as

$$E[(Y_1 - Y_2)^2] = (\mu_1 - \mu_2)^2 + (\sigma_1 - \sigma_2)^2 + 2(1 - \rho)\sigma_1\sigma_2$$

The CCC is then defined as a scaleless index ρ_c:

$$\rho_c = 1 - \frac{E[(Y_1 - Y_2)^2]}{\sigma_1^2 + \sigma_2^2 + (\mu_1 - \mu_2)^2} \tag{2.12}$$

Equivalently, ρ_c can be written as

$$\rho_c = \frac{2\rho\sigma_1\sigma_2}{\sigma_1^2 + \sigma_2^2 + (\mu_1 - \mu_2)^2} \tag{2.13}$$

Therefore, ρ_c is different from ρ by a factor of $\frac{2\sigma_1\sigma_2}{\sigma_1^2 + \sigma_2^2 + (\mu_1 - \mu_2)^2}$. For n independent pair of sample data, ρ_c is estimated by its sample counterpart, i.e.,

$$\hat{\rho}_c = \frac{2s_{12}}{s_1^2 + s_2^2 + (\bar{y}_1 - \bar{y}_2)^2}$$

where $\bar{y}_j = \sum_{i=1}^n y_{ij}/n, s_j^2 = \sum_{i=1}^n (y_{ij} - \bar{y}_j)^2/n$ for $j = 1, 2$; and $s_{12} = \sum_{i=1}^n (y_{i1} - \bar{y}_1)(y_{i2} - \bar{y}_2)/n$. Note that the factor $\frac{1}{n}$ in the sample variances s_1^2, s_2^2 and sample covariance s_{12} are better replaced by $\frac{1}{n-1}$ to have unbiased estimations. The more ρ_c is close to 1, the more the pair of sample measurements from two labs can be concluded to be in agreement. As suggested in Lin (1992), a least acceptable bound can be computed. If the 95% lower bound of Lin's CCC is above the least acceptable bound, then measurements from the two labs are concordant.

One caveat of using Lin's CCC is that the population under consideration should be relatively hetergeneous, meaning that the measurement range should be larger than the within-subject variability. In other words, Lin's CCC is sensitive to population heterogeneity or subject-to-subject variability. This has been cautioned by several researchers. For instance, Atkinson and Nevill (1997) illustrated this effect by considering the following example shown in Table 2.6. In this example, data (1) and data (2) have a different spread of measurements, but the pairwise differences are exactly the same. However, data (1) has CCC of 0.78, demonstrating some degree of agreement and data (2) has a very low CCC of 0.28, showing little agreement of the two tests.

TABLE 2.6
Two data sets with different between-subject variability but have same degree
of agreement as measured by the limits of agreement of Bland-Altman method.
Source: Atkinson and Nevill (1997).

	Data Set 1			Data Set 2	
Test 1	Test 2	Difference	Test 1	Test 2	Difference
31	27	-4	41	37	-4
33	35	2	43	45	2
42	47	5	42	47	5
40	44	4	40	44	4
63	63	0	43	43	0
28	31	3	48	51	3
43	54	11	43	54	11
44	54	10	44	54	10
68	68	0	48	48	0
47	58	11	47	58	11
47	48	1	47	48	1
40	43	3	40	43	3
43	45	2	43	45	2
47	52	5	47	52	5
58	48	-10	58	48	-10
61	61	0	41	41	0
45	52	7	45	52	7
43	44	1	43	44	1
58	48	-10	58	48	-10
40	44	4	40	44	4
48	47	-1	48	47	-1
42	52	10	42	52	10
61	45	-16	61	45	-16
48	43	-5	48	43	-5
43	52	9	43	52	9
50	52	2	50	52	2
39	40	1	39	40	1
52	58	6	52	58	6
42	45	3	42	45	3
77	67	-10	57	47	-10
Mean					
47.4	48.9	1.5	46.1	47.6	1.5
SD					
10.9	9.4	6.6	5.9	5.1	6.6

As recommended by Atkinson and Nevill (1997), an alternative measure of agreement by Bland and Altman (Bland and Altman (1986, 1999)) may be more appropriate. The Bland–Altman method is based on the pairwise difference of the same samples tested in both laboratories. Assuming normality assumption, the pairwise difference has mean d and variance σ_d^2, then the 95% limits of agreement can be obtained as $\overline{d} + / - 1.96 s_d$. If these limits are within the acceptable ranges as determined by subject matter experts, then the two laboratories are considered to be in agreement. In addition, the confidence limits for the mean difference can also be constructed to detect if there is any bias. A graphical presentation of the Bland–Altman method is perhaps more intuitive. As shown in Figure 2.13, instead of presenting the raw data in the graph with a reference line of 45 degree with intercept 0 and slope 1, the Bland-Altman plot has the difference as y-axis and the average as x-axis. By presenting the data in this way, the variability of the difference can be shown more clearly, and the limits of agreement can also be imposed. If the variability of difference is not constant and shows some pattern instead, then appropriate transformation on the difference may be taken to stabilize the variance. Logarithm is the common transformation to be taken. Several alternative methods have been proposed in the past decades, such as Lin's (Lin (2000)) total deviation index (TDI), Zhong et al.'s tolerance interval approach (Zhong et al. (2008)), Barnhart et al.'s coefficient of individual agreement (CIA) (Barnhart et al. (2007)), to name a few.

The quasi-quantitative nature of immunogenicity assay makes the choice of statistical methods rather challenging. Some may argue that the criteria of measuring individual agreement used for quantitative data may be too stringent for immunogenicity data. After all, it is the positive-negative classification that matters, not the absolute value of the signal readout. The Kappa coefficient (Landis and Koch (1977)) used to assess agreement of nominal scale may be more appropriate, as was utilized in Tatarewicz et al. (2009).

In the third step, Tatarewicz et al. (2009) proposed to have performance testing using the process involved in clinical sample tests; see Tatarewicz et al. (2009) for details.

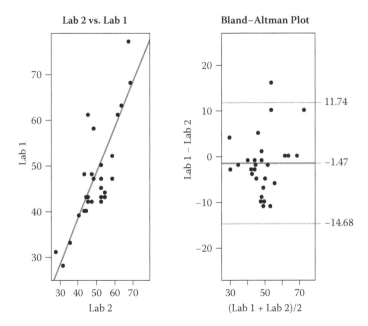

FIGURE 2.13
Plot of data from Lab 1 versus Lab 2. feft: scatter plot with 45 degree reference
line. right: Bland–Altman plot with limits of agreement imposed.

3

Determination of ADA Assay Cut Point

CONTENTS

3.1 Introduction

As demonstrated in the previous chapter, the key assay performance parameters during assay validation are the cut points for screening, confirmatory, and neutralizing assays. Due to the product-, process-, and patient-related factors that can contribute to the variability of immunogenicity data, determination of cut point is not straightforward. According to regulatory guidances and white papers FDA (2009), USP<1106>, and Shankar et al. (2008), cut points should be statistically derived from data generated during pre-study validation. According to Shankar et al. (2008), for the screening assay validation, typically 50 samples are needed for the screening cut point determination. The experimental design for the establishment of cut point is described in section 3.2. In section 3.3, statistical details for the determination of cut points are introduced, with an emphasis on screening cut point determination. The "white paper" approach by Shankar et al. (2008) will be introduced followed by some recent advancements in research community on cut point determination.

3.2   Cut Point Experimental Design

It is well known that immunogenicity data are subject to heterogeneity of sample population as well as variability associated with assay itself. One objective of assay validation is to understand these variabilities. Correctly identifying these variance components and reducing potential effects of confounding factors are important for setting a cut point that maintains the targeted false positive rate. For example, if analyst 1 uses instrument 1 to test all the samples and these samples are also tested by analyst 2 using instrument 2, the source of the variability (i.e., analyst, instrument, or both) cannot be determined. Likewise, Zhong and Zhou (2013) argued that if the samples are grouped into three subsets and only one subset of samples is tested by each analyst, it is difficult to attribute the variability to analyst or to the sample grouping. Similar examples were illustrated by Devanarayan and Tovey (2011). To this end, balanced experimental designs are recommended to better estimate variance components (Shankar et al. (2008)). Figure 3.1 contains an example of a balanced experiment design. In this example, 48 donors are randomly allocated to three groups. Additionally, all samples are tested on three different plates.[1]

Statistically, the following model can be used to estimate the variance components:

$$Y_{ijkl} = \mu + d_i + \alpha_j + \beta_{k(j)} + \tau_l + \epsilon_{ijkl} \tag{3.1}$$

where Y_{ijkl} refers to the ith donor signal reading from jth analyst at kth run and on the lth plate. d_i, α_j, $\beta_{k(j)}$, τ_l are independently and normally distributed with mean 0 and variance σ_d^2, σ_α^2, σ_β^2, σ_τ^2, respectively, representing the donor-to-donor, analyst-to-analyst, run-to-run, and plate-to-plate variability. ϵ_{ijkl} is the error term with mean 0 and variance σ^2. The model can be modified to include fixed effects, if any. The variance components can be estimated using a random effect ANOVA model. Table 3.1 is a numerical example. In this example, the analyst-to-analyst variability and possibly plate-to-plate variability are significant and can not be neglected.

Careful consideration of cut point design is therefore important to identify key variability contributors and reduce the impact of uncontrollable factors. With the assistance of a statistician, statistical analyses can be used to improve the quality of the data used for cut point.

Ideally, cut points should be determined from data generated from samples of drug-naive donors from the target disease population. However, in some

---

[1]This is a Latin-square design with respect to runs and plates for each analyst.

		Subject Grouping		
	Run	S1-S16	S17-S32	S33-S48
Analyst 1	1	Plate 1	Plate 2	Plate 3
	2	Plate 3	Plate 1	Plate 2
	3	Plate 2	Plate 3	Plate 1
Analyst 2	1	Plate 1	Plate 2	Plate 3
	2	Plate 3	Plate 1	Plate 2
	3	Plate 2	Plate 3	Plate 1

FIGURE 3.1
Example of balanced design for cut point.

TABLE 3.1
A numerical example of variance components analysis

Source of Variability	Variance Estimate	Percent of Total
Donor	0.0203	66.56
Analyst	0.0062	20.33
Run(Analyst)	0.0003	0.98
Assay Plate	0.0032	10.49
Residual	0.0005	1.64
Total	0.0305	100

cases, it may not be possible to obtain enough donors of certain diseases. Consequently, healthy donors are often used to establish the initial cut point; and adjustment may be made based on the availability of diseased donors. Healthy donors are also used for some Phase I clinical studies where normal volunteers are recruited. The validity of such cut point should be closely monitored and re-established if the existing cut point is demonstrated to be inadequate. Sometimes, several disease indications are under investigation at the same time. In this case, it is expected that an equal number of donors from each disease indication are tested. Distributions of assay responses should be compared among the different disease indications. Depending on the distributions, a common cut point or disease-specific cut points may be warranted.

One question that scientists often ask is: How many donors are needed? According to Shankar et al. (2008) and USP<1106>, more than 50 donors are needed to obtain cut point for robust evaluation in clinical studies. For nonclinical studies, 15 to 30 donors are recommended (USP<1106>). While justifications for the recommended sample numbers were not provided, it is well understood that reliable cut point determination requires either more donors or more replicates for each donor. Statistical analyses are useful to determine what sample size (of donors and/or replications) is appropriate. In hypothesis testing, the problem of sample size is well-defined and is based on type-I and type-II errors (or power). Although power calculation is frequently used for sample size planning, criterion based on precision of cut point estimator is more appropriate in the situation of cut point determination. Similar to hypothesis testing, the sample size is dependent on the underlying statistical distribution. Zhang et al. (2014) considered the sample size problem for ADA screening cut point. The cut point in their work is based on one-way and two-way random effect models under normal assumption. In particular, they consider the following models, namely,

$$Y_{ij} = \mu + d_i + \epsilon_{ij} \tag{3.2}$$

and

$$Y_{ij} = \mu + d_i + \beta_j + \epsilon_{ij} \tag{3.3}$$

where Y_{ij} is the normalized assay response from the ith donor in the jth run of a cut point experiment. μ is the grand mean, d_i is the random effect of the ith donor, β_j (if in the model) is the random effect of the jth run, and the error term ϵ_{ij} accounts for the remaining variability for the ith donor in the jth run. For a cut point estimator $\hat{q}_p$ at false positive rate p, Zhang et al. (2014) proposed to use precision as the criteria and define the precision of cut point estimator as

$$D = \frac{\sigma(\hat{q}_p)}{q_p} \tag{3.4}$$

where $\sigma(\hat{q})$ refers to the standard error of $\hat{q}_p$. This definition is motivated by several authors, e.g., Bonett (2002) who used confidence-interval width as a precision criteria for sample size planning. In a similar situation of quantile estimation, Garsd et al. (1983) defines the precision d such that

$$Pr(|X_{p,n} - q_p| \geq dq_p) = \alpha, \tag{3.5}$$

where $X_{p,n}$ is the $100p$th sample quantile. By asymptotic normality theory, the relationship between D and d is approximately

$$d = z_{1-\alpha}D, \tag{3.6}$$

where $z_{1-\alpha}$ is the $100(1-\alpha)$th quantile of standard normal distribution. Intuitively, d can be interpreted as the ratio of half-width of the $100(1-\alpha)$ confidence interval for q_α to itself, or the half-width of the $100(1-\alpha)$ confidence interval for q_p on the relative scale. Hence, for example, when $D = 0.04$ and $\alpha = 5\%$, we are about 95% confident that the estimate of q_p will be approximately within the range of -8% and 8% of q_p. The precision involves the number of donors and number of replicates, and thus can be used to determine the minimal required sample size. Because the effect of bias of cut point estimate in models (3.2) and (3.3) is negligible, it is sufficient to use precision only. For a desired precision, say, $D_0 = 0.05$, the minimal required sample size can be calculated by finding the solution to the following inequality:

$$\arg\min_{I} \left\{ \hat{D} = \frac{\hat{\sigma}(\hat{q}_p)}{\hat{q}_p} \geq D_0 \right\} \tag{3.7}$$

while assuming the number of replicates for each donor is the same and kept fixed. $\hat{D}$ is the estimation of D by replacing the unknown quantities in D with their corresponding estimates. In addition, the calculation of sample size requires the preliminary inputs of μ, σ_d and σ_e of model (3.2) or (3.3). Table 3.2 gives the calculated minimal sample size for fixed number of replicates in various scenarios for model (3.2).

From Table 3.2, it is seen that the relative magnitude of the mean and the total variability as well as intraclass correlation coefficient (the ratio of the between-donor variability versus total variability) have immense impact on the required sample size to achieve the same level of precision for the cut point estimator. Overall, larger total variability (relative to mean) requires a larger sample size. For the same total variability, larger intraclass correlation coefficient requires a larger sample size. Generally, increasing number of replicates does not have much effect on reducing the sample size when the intraclass correlation coefficient is relatively large; see Zhang et al. (2014) for more details.

The criterion used for sample size calculation is reasonable from a statistical perspective but it is perhaps more sensible to have similar criterion in terms of false positive rate. In addition, the above results are based on models assuming normal distribution. Non-normal distributions generally require larger sample sizes than those of normal distributions. Therefore, the results under the normal distribution can be considered to be the minimal sample size needed for cut point experiment planning.

3.3   Statistical Methods for Cut Point Determination

As described in Chapter 2, immunogenicity is typically evaluated using a tiered approach consisting of a screening assay followed by a confirmatory assay and additional characterization steps. Determination of cut points are thus critical to the immunogenicity assays. In this section, the statistical procedure of cut point determination is described, mainly from the work by Shankar et al. (2008). This method is frequently used by industry for cut point determination. Because of this, the method is referred to as the "white paper" approach for convenience. However, the method is not perfect, and cut point determination continues to be an active research area. In this section, some recent developments in the literature are also introduced.

TABLE 3.2
The minimal required sample size to meet the 0.05 precision for different intraclass correlation and different number of replicates. The three panels (upper, middle and bottom) are corresponding to three different scenarios: (a) mean=1.0,variance=0.1; (b) mean=1.2, varaince=0.1; (c) mean=1.0, variance=0.01.

ρ	J=2	J=4	J=6	J=8
0.1	22	12	9	7
0.3	25	16	14	12
0.5	29	22	20	19
0.7	33	29	27	27
0.8	36	33	32	31
0.9	39	37	37	36
0.95	40	39	39	39
0.99	41	41	41	41

ρ	J=2	J=4	J=6	J=8
0.1	17	10	7	6
0.3	20	13	11	10
0.5	22	17	16	15
0.7	26	23	22	21
0.8	28	26	25	25
0.9	30	29	29	29
0.95	32	31	31	31
0.99	32	32	32	32

ρ	J=2	J=4	J=6	J=8
0.1	4	3	2	2
0.3	5	4	3	3
0.5	6	5	4	4
0.7	6	5	5	5
0.8	7	6	6	6
0.9	7	7	7	7
0.95	8	7	7	7
0.99	8	8	8	8

3.3.1   White Paper Approach

The "white paper" approach has been described in detail in the appendix in Shankar et al. (2008) and further explained in Devanarayan and Tovey (2011). Cut point is typically established during the validation study and applied to in-study samples. Depending on the nature of cut point data, there are three types of screening cut points, namely, (a) fixed cut point;(b) floating cut point; and (c) dynamic cut point. The fixed cut point is calculated based on raw validation assay signal readouts and directly compared with samples to declare sample positivity. The floating cut point is a value obtained by applying a normalization factor, determined from the validation data, to the background value during the in-study stage. In other words, the normalization factor can be considered fixed from validation stage to in-study stage and it may be called cut point factor. Dynamic cut point is a cut point which may change from instrument to instrument or from analyst to analyst. An investigation is warranted in such situation. Consequently, an analyst-specific or instrument-specific fixed or floating cut point may be used. In an AAPS survey by Gorovits (2009), many biopharmaceutical companies reported to use floating cut points. In the following, we will focus on the floating cut point. According to Shankar et al. (2008), the process of determining the screening cut point consists of several steps: (1) investigate the distribution and exclude outliers; (2) compare assay run means and variances to determine which type of cut point is appropriate; and (3) calculate the screening cut point. A schematic diagram is presented in Figure 3.2.

3.3.1.1 Investigate Distribution and Exclude Outliers

The first step is to determine the distribution of the data. If the data have a non-normal distribution, then an appropriate method of data transformation such as logarithmic transformation is chosen. The purpose of selection of an appropriate transformation is based on the intuition that the data would be more symmetric and closer to a normal distribution on the transformed scale. The skewness parameter may be estimated from the data; the Shapiro–Wilk (Shapiro and Wilk (1965)) normality test is also performed to assess the normality of the data. If the skewness parameter and p-value from the normality test indicate that the data under logarithmic transformation are more symmetric and more normal, which is typically the case, the logarithmic transformation should be taken on all the data values. Devanarayan and Tovey (2011) recommended that the selection of transformation be based on averaged data (with respect to donor) across all the runs. A more reasonable approach is to consider the Box–Cox (Box and Cox (1964)) transformation. It is a rank-preserving transformation, which means that relative order of the data values are kept the same on the transformed scale as on the original scale. The Box–Cox transformation is a family of transformations controlled by a parameter λ. It has the form:

$$h(y) = \begin{cases} \frac{y^{\lambda}-1}{\lambda}, & \text{if } \lambda \neq 0. \\ \log(y), & \text{if } \lambda = 0. \end{cases} \tag{3.8}$$

The Box–Cox procedure automatically identifies a transformation through the maximum likelihood estimation (MLE) of parameter λ to find the most appropriate transformation for correcting skewness of the distribution.

Once appropriate transformation is determined, all subsequent analyses of data, such as outlier evaluation, comparison of means and variances among

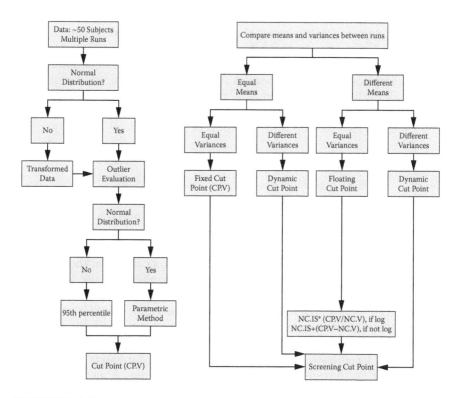

FIGURE 3.2

A schematic diagram for screening cut point determination. NC.V: Negative control for validation runs. NC.IS: Negative control for in-study runs. Modified from Figure 1 of Shankar et al. (2008).

assay runs and cut point calculation should be performed on the transformed scale. After the data has been transformed, outliers should be removed before determining the cut point. Shankar et al. (2008) does not distinguish different type of outliers. Devanarayan and Tovey (2011), however, define two types of outliers known as biological outliers and analytical outliers. Biological outliers are outliers due to the heterogeneity of the donor/sample population. For example, some pre-existing antibodies manifest extremely high signals and would be presumably flagged by outlier removal procedures. For the same donor or sample, some value from one run may be extremely higher or lower than the values from the other runs. Such value may be suspected as analytical outlier. The existence of biological outliers or an analytical outliers inflates the biological and assay variability (in addition to affect the mean or median), respectively, consequently inflating the cut point estimation and deflating false positive rate. Therefore, it is expected that these outliers should be removed before cut point calculations. However, the identification of outliers is not a trivial task. Devanarayan and Tovey (2011) recommended that Tukey's box-plot method be used for outlier identification. Specifically, they recommended that the outlier boxplot criteria to be used to analyze the distribution of data from each assay run as well we the average data values across the assay runs. Outliers from the average of the data are biological outliers while outliers identified from each assay run are analytical outliers. Zhang et al. (2013) demonstrated that the analytical outliers should be removed before the biological outliers. This is because, for any donor, the analytical outlier is relative to that donor's own mean signal level. The boxplot criterion applying to each assay run clearly involves both biological variability and analytical variability. Consequently, the donor average value may be distorted due to some extremely high or low analytical outliers.

3.3.1.2 Compare Assay Run Means and Variances

The "white paper" recommends conducting an ANOVA and testing the equality of assay run means as well as the homogeneity of variances across assay runs. The selection of which type of cut point to use depends on the test result. If the assay run means and variances are not statistically different, the fixed cut point may be used; the floating cut point can be also used in this case. If the assay run means are statistically different, but the variances are not statistically different, the floating cut point can be used. When assay variances are statistically different, the dynamic cut point may be used. In the last case, an investigation is warranted. To test mean equality and variance homogeneity, consider the ANOVA model:

$$Y_{ij} = \mu + \beta_j + \epsilon_{ij} \tag{3.9}$$

where Y_{ij} denotes the transformed assay signal of the ith donor at jth run, β_j denotes the effect of the jth run, and ϵ_{ij} denotes the normally distributed error of the ith donor at jth run with mean 0 and variance σ^2. Assume there are I donors in total with each being assayed for J runs, resulting in $N = IJ$ signal readouts in total. To test the equality of run means that β_js equal 0, the ANOVA F-test can be used. The ANOVA table is shown in Table 3.3.

TABLE 3.3
ANOVA table for testing assay run means

Source	SS	DF	MS	EMS
Inter-run	$SSA = I\sum_j(\overline{y}_{.j} - \overline{y})^2$	$J-1$	MSA	$\sigma^2 + \frac{I\sum \beta_j^2}{J-1}$
Intra-run	$SSE = \sum_{i,j}(y_{ij} - \overline{y}_{.j})^2$	$(I-1)J$	MSE	σ^2
Total	$SSTO = \sum_{i,j}(y_{ij} - \overline{y})^2$	$IJ-1$		

where $MSA = SSA/(J-1)$, $MSE = SSE/((I-1)J)$.

The F-test statistic is the ratio of MSA versus MSE. As their expectations indicate, when β_js are equal, the F ratio is close to 1. When the run means are equal, the F-test statistic follows an F distribution with $J-1$ and $N-J$ degrees of freedom. To test if the J runs of data have equal variances, Bartlett's test (Snedecor and Cochran (1989)) can be applied. However, Bartlett's test is reportedly to be sensitive to normality assumption. A more robust test is Levene's test (Levene (1960)). Levene's test is often used before a comparison of means. Let $z_{ij} = |y_{ij} - \overline{y}_{.j}|$ be the absolute deviations. Levene's test determines whether the expected values of the absolute deviations for the J runs are equal. The Brown–Forsythe test (Brown and Forsythe (1974)) modified Levene's test by replacing the mean with median to have a more robust test against many types of non-normality while retaining good statistical power. Levene's test or Brown–Forsythe test statistic is simply the F test statistic used to test equality of means by replacing y_{ij} with z_{ij}. The resulting test statistic approximately follows an F distribution with the same degrees of freedom. Brown and Forsythe (1974) performed Monte Carlo simulation studies which indicate that using the trimmed mean performed best when the underlying data followed a Cauchy distribution (a heavy-tailed distribution) and the median performed best when the underlying data followed a χ^2 distribution with four degrees of freedom (a heavily skewed distribution). The mean based Levene's test provides the best power for symmetric, moderate-tailed distributions.

3.3.1.3 Calculate the Screening Cut Point

Depending on the distribution of the data, a parametric method or non-parametric method may be used to determine the screening cut point. As an alternative to the parametric method, the robust method can be used as it is robust against outliers and the assumption of normality. The robust method estimates the center and spread using the median instead of the mean and the median absolute deviation (MAD) instead of the standard deviation. The

MAD is defined as

$$MAD = \texttt{median}\{y_i - \tilde{y}\}$$

where $\tilde{y}$ is the median. If the data are normally distributed, then it can be shown that $E[1.483 \times MAD] = \sigma$, the standard deviation of normal distribution. If the data appear to be normally distributed after transformation and outlier removal, the parametric method can be used. A simple procedure would be to estimate the standard deviation from each run and then pool them. The method of averaging the results across all the runs for each donor is discouraged as it neglects the intra-assay variability and consequently will underestimate the true cut point. Formally, the mean and standard deviation can be estimated from the ANOVA model mentioned above. The screening cut point is then calculated as $mean + 1.645 \times SD$. For robust method, the median and $1.483 \times MAD$, play the roles of mean and standard deviation. A more rigorous way is the mixed-effect ANOVA model (3.3):

$$Y_{ij} = \mu + d_i + \beta_j + \epsilon_{ij} \tag{3.10}$$

The screening cut point is then calculated as $mean + 1.645 \times SD$. The standard deviation here refers to the total variability which incorporates both the inter-donor variability (biological variability) and intra-assay variability (analytical variability). If the normality assumption is violated, the nonparametric approach is often used. The 95th percentile/quantile is calculated accordingly. For floating cut point, the cut point factor is determined by subtracting the average of negative control across the runs from the estimated cut point. The floating cut point for an in-study assay is then the run mean of the negative control plus the cut point factor. If the log-transformation is applied, the cut point factor is obtained by dividing the floating cut point by the average of negative control and the in-study cut point is the product of the cut point factor and the average of the negative control of the in-study assay run. For other transformation other than log-transformation, the cut point factor may be obtained by subtracting the average of the negative control from the cut point on that transformed scale before transforming back to the original scale.

One caveat of determining floating cut point is that, for the cut point factor to be constant across the runs, the run-specific negative control should be able to correct for the run-to-run deviation. In other words, the negative control background-corrected signal should behave similarly as the uncorrected signal in the fixed cut point case. The underlying assumption for the floating cut point is that the negative control background-corrected individual sample distribution should behave similarly across all the runs. While this assumption may be hard to verify, Devanarayan and Tovey (2011) proposed to check the correlation or linear relationship of the negative controls average from each of the assay runs versus the average of the individual donor samples from the corresponding runs.

For neutralizing assay, Gupta et al. (2011) recommended similar method for calculating neutralizing screening cut point. If there is no additional assay to eliminate false positive classifications, a false positive rate of 1% is recommended.

3.3.1.4   Confirmatory Cut Point

A confirmatory cut point in the second tier of immunogenicity testing is used to distinguish between specific and nonspecific binding activities and eliminate the latter. In the "white paper" approach, the inhibition data for each donor are generated on the same plate as the screening cut point data by analyzing the same drug-naïve samples in presence and absence of excess drug. The signal change upon addition of drug is usually expressed as %Inhibition:

$$\%Inhibition = 100 \times \left[1 - \frac{\texttt{Signal in Presence of Drug}}{\texttt{Signal in Absence of Drug}} \right] \qquad (3.11)$$

The %Inhibition values can be negative and thus not amenable to logarithmic transformation. For this reason, Kubiak et al. (2013) argued that the ratio of signal in absence of drug to signal in presence of drug may be preferred for use in statistical analyse. Kubiak et al. (2013) defines the inhibition ratio or IR as:

$$IR = \frac{\texttt{Signal in Absence of Drug}}{\texttt{Signal in Presence of Drug}} \qquad (3.12)$$

The IR values are always positive, can be subjected to log-transformation and is more suitable for analysis of intra- and inter-assay precision.

The confirmatory cut point used to eliminate false positive samples detected from screening assay should also be statistically derived from the data distribution of same samples used for screening cut point experiment, due to the lack of true positive samples during the validation stage. Calculation of a confirmatory cut point is similar to that of the fixed screening cut point. Appropriate transformation and outlier removal is recommended. Interestingly, many inhibition data sets demonstrate nearly normal distribution after outlier removal, according to the authors' personal experience. If transformation is not possible due to negative values of %Inhibition, IR can be used instead. A confirmatory false positive rate of 1% or 0.1% is recommended by Shankar et al. (2008).

3.3.2   Some Recent Developments

While the approach recommended by the "white paper" is very detailed and easy to follow for practitioners, with the assistance of statistician whenever possible, there are still some aspects that are currently being discussed in the literature and can be improved in practice.

3.3.2.1   Data Normalization

Zhang et al. (2013) argued that using the ANOVA model (3.9) with run factor only to determine which type of cut point to use is discouraged since an insignificant result may be due to the large biological variability, and a significant result may be due to the relative large sample size of donors. As a result, they suggested using the floating cut point. In addition, they recommended that the raw individual data should be normalized by dividing the average of the negative control on that plate. Compared with the data without normalization, the run-to-run variability after data normalization is reduced dramatically without diminishing the donor-to-donor variability. For this reason, Zhang et al. (2013) recommended using the floating cut point based on normalized data. A random-effect model such as model (3.2) can be used to determine the cut point with the assistance of a statistician. If the data are normally distributed, the resulting cut point is calculated as $mean + 1.645 \times sqrt(\texttt{total variability})$. Alternatively, one can pool all the data from all the runs together and determine the cut point without considering the data structure. This seems counter-intuitive and leads to biased estimate of cut point. However, such bias is very small as demonstrated by Zhang et al. (2013) if the data are normally distributed. Separately, Hutson (2003) demonstrated that similar conclusion can be made for the non-parametric method. This result gives scientists great flexibility to perform the analysis by themselves. However, the impact of variance of cut point estimator should also be evaluated if such variance needs to be reported along with the cut point. It is conjectured that the variance assuming the pooled data are independent would be underestimated greatly.

3.3.2.2 Outliers

Shankar et al. (2008) mentioned that the boxplot method can be used for outlier detection. However, it is not clear how to identify biological outliers and analytical outliers. Devanarayan and Tovey (2011) described the procedure as follows: (1) calculate the average value across all the runs for each donor; (2) apply the boxplot method to the sample means and remove those donors whose means are beyond the boxplot fences[2]; (3) after removing all donors identified from (2), apply boxplot method for each run and remove values outside the fences. Donors identified and excluded in step (2) are considered biological outliers and values identified in step (3) are analytical outliers. This approach is very easy to implement. However, Zhang et al. (2013) showed that the approach cannot identify the outliers correctly. They considered the following hypothetical scenario. Suppose 48 donors were tested in four runs and the data are shown in the upper left panel in Figure 3.3. Now assume that due to a recording error, the signal readings from donor 1 and donor 2 in run 2 were switched by mistake(lower left panel in Figure 3.3). As a result, these two values from donor 1 and 2 in run 2 were considerably different from value of the same donor from other runs and should be detected as analytical outliers. Now follow the above procedure and apply the boxplot method to donor averages (upper right panel in Figure 3.3). Two separate donors were identified as

---

[2]Any data points beyond the boxplot fences are considered outliers.

biological outliers and all values of these two donors were then removed. Next, apply the boxplot method to each run of the remaining data (lower right panel in Figure 3.3), the two analytical outliers in run 2 were well within the fences and not flagged out. The reason is that analytical outlier should be detected based on analytical variability by separating the biological variability out. Zhang et al. (2013) argued that analytical outliers should be detected before biological outliers. Using model (3.2), the residuals from the model can be used for detecting analytical outliers and the predicted donor values can be used to detect biological outliers. The second approach as recommended by Zhang et al. (2013) would first detect analytical outliers by looking at data donor by donor, then the donor averages are subject to biological outlier detection. In summary, a simplified version of cut point determination procedure as shown in Figure 3.4 can be implemented by scientists directly with the help of some statistical softwares.

In practice, removing significant amount of data, especially biological outliers, is often found to be undesirable with the consequence of low cut point and high ADA incidence rate found in clinical studies. Therefore, removing biological outliers should be extremely careful. Currently, there is no consensus on whether and how to remove biological outliers.

3.3.2.3   Non-Normal Distributions

Oftentimes, the data is not normally distributed and an appropriate transformation may not be readily available. In addition, many immune response data of screening assay appear to be unimodal and skewed to the right. Motivated by these, Schlain et al. (2010) proposed to use a three-parameter gamma distribution to fit cut point data. The three-parametric gamma density function is:

$$f(x) = \frac{(x-\tau)^{\eta-1}\exp\left[-(x-\tau)/\theta\right]}{\theta^\eta\Gamma(\eta)}, \quad \eta > 0, \theta > 0, x > \tau \qquad (3.13)$$

where η is the shape parameter, θ is the scale parameter and τ is the threshold parameter. When the shape parameter η goes to infinity, the gamma distribution degenerates to a normal distribution; see Figure 3.5 for the density plot. The method of MLE may be used to obtain parameter estimation through numerical iteration since closed-form solution is usually not available. Given the data of n independent random variables $x_1, x_2, \cdots, x_n$, each distributed as in (3.13), the MLE of parameter can be obtained by solving the following

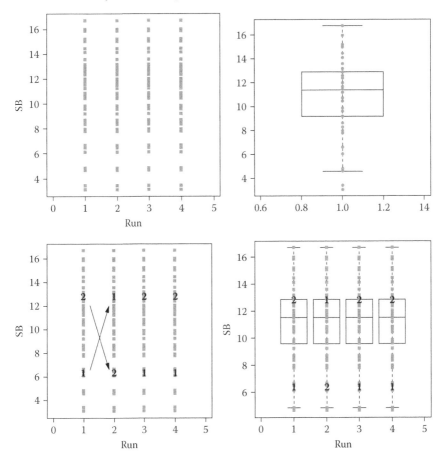

FIGURE 3.3
Illustration of impact of outliers removal order. Source: Zhang et al. (2013)

equations:

$$\sum_{i=1}^{n} \log(x_i - \hat{\tau}) - n \log \hat{\theta} - n\psi(\eta) = 0$$

$$\sum_{i=1}^{n} (x_i - \hat{\tau}) - n\hat{\eta}\hat{\theta} = 0$$

$$-\sum_{i=1}^{n} (x_i - \hat{\tau})^{-1} + n\{\hat{\theta}(\hat{\eta} - 1)\} = 0$$

where $\hat{\eta}, \hat{\theta}, \hat{\tau}$ stand for MLE for η, θ, τ, respectively. However, it is noted that when the shape parameter η is close to 1, the MLE is unstable and thus not

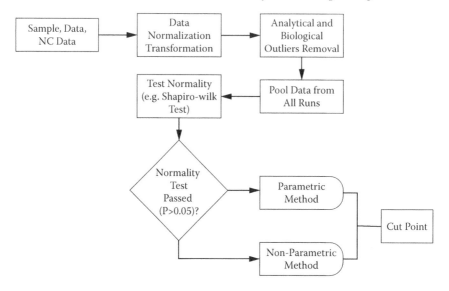

FIGURE 3.4
A flow chart for cut point determination. Source: Zhang et al. (2013)

recommended. If the method of moment is used, the estimators $\tilde{\eta}, \tilde{\theta}, \tilde{\tau}$ satisfy the following equations:

$$\tilde{\tau} + \tilde{\eta}\tilde{\theta} = \overline{x}$$
$$\tilde{\eta}\tilde{\theta}^2 = \mu_2$$
$$2\tilde{\eta}\tilde{\theta}^3 = \mu_3$$

where $\mu_2 = \sum(x_i - \overline{x})^2/n, \mu_3 = \sum(x_i - \overline{x})^3/n$ are the second and third central moments, respectively. Although the method of moments estimators can be solved from the above equations explicitly, it can be shown that, for example, the variance of $\tilde{\eta}$ is substantially larger than $\hat{\eta}$. Given that the method of moment estimation is less precise than the MLE, Whitten and Cohen (1986) recommended using the modified moment estimation (MME) when the shape parameter $\eta < 1.78$. In MME, the central third moment μ_3 is replaced by the expectation of cumulative distribution function of the minimal order statistics, such that $E[F(X_{(1)})] = 1/(n+1)$. For extensive discussion of gamma distribution in general and its parameter estimation, see Johnson et al. (1994).

The lognormal distribution is also unimodal and skewed to right. If X follows a normal distribution with mean μ and variance σ^2, then $Y = \exp(X)$ follows lognormal distribution; see Figure 3.6 for the density plot. It is noted that, for the lognormal distribution as defined above, the mean is $\exp\{\mu + \sigma^2/2\}$, the median is $\exp\{\mu\}$, and the variance is $\exp\{2\mu + \sigma^2/2\} * (\exp\{\sigma^2\} -$

Density of Gamma Distribution

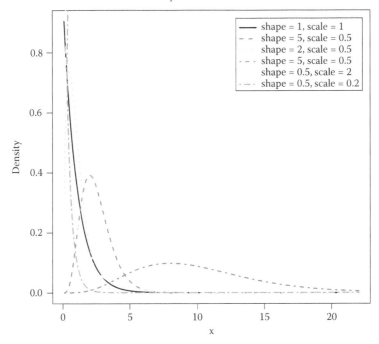

FIGURE 3.5
Density of gamma distribution with various shape and scale (threshold is set at 0).

1). Parameter estimation is straightforward since the log-transformed data is normally distributed.

Simulation studies reported by Schlain et al. (2010) showed that if the data follow the gamma distribution, the method based on normal distribution can over-estimate the false positive rate (with the target of 5%) by as much as 3%. On the other hand, if the data follow lognormal distribution, it could deviate downward by as large as 2.3% on average. The non-parametric method has much more variability than that of gamma distribution when the sample size is small. It could inflate the false positive rate by as much as 2.5% for small sample size. With moderate sample size, the loss of efficiency of nonparametric method depends on the specific underlying true distribution. Therefore, the impact on false positive rate should be evaluated case-by-case.

One disadvantage of gamma or lognormal distribution is that it does not take repeated-measures data structure into account unless the gamma or log-

Density of Lognormal Distribution

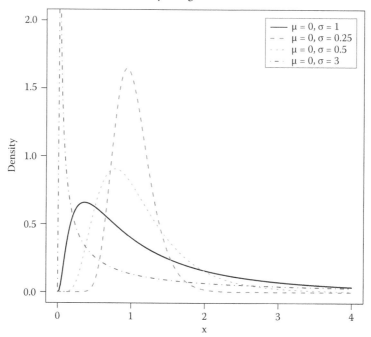

FIGURE 3.6
Density of lognormal distribution with location and scale.

normal distribution are fitted to the data from each run, and the run-wise cut points are summarized to obtain a final cut point. Alternatively, models directly taking data structure into account can be considered. Zhang et al. (2015) considered non-normal random effect models. They proposed the following non-normal random effect model:

$$y_{ij} = \mu + b_i + \epsilon_{ij} \qquad (3.14)$$

where $\mu + b_i$ represents the unknown mean response of donor i and is assumed to be random. Instead of considering the usual variance components model where b_i are normally distributed, Zhang et al. (2015) proposed to use non-normal distribution for b_i, which is demonstrated by screening assay data. In particular, they considered two non-normal distributions, namely, the skew-t distribution and log-gamma distribution. The Student t-distribution as well as the skew-t distribution are robust to outliers by downweighting the extreme data values. In addition, it has heavier tail than the normal distribution.

The skew-t distribution was originally proposed by Azzalini and Capitanio (2003) and Sahu et al. (2003) separately. Following Sahu et al. (2003), a skew-t random variable X has the density function of the following form:

$$f(x|\mu, \sigma^2, \delta, \nu) = 2t_\nu(x|\mu, \sigma^2 + \delta^2)T_{\nu+1}\left(\frac{\delta}{\sigma}\frac{x-\mu}{\sqrt{\sigma^2+\delta^2}}\left\{\frac{\nu + q(x,\mu)}{\nu+1}\right\}^{-1/2}\right)$$
(3.15)

where $t_m(\cdot|\mu, s^2)$ denotes the univariate Student t-distribution with location parameter μ, scale parameter s and degree of freedom m; $T_m(\cdot)$ represents the corresponding cumulative distribution function with location 0, scale 1 and degree of freedom m. $q(x,\mu) = (x - \mu)(\sigma^2 + \delta^2)^{-1}(x - \mu)$ denotes the Mahalanobis distance between x and μ. We denote the skew-t distribution by $ST_\nu(\mu, \sigma, \delta)$. The mean and variance are $E(X) = \mu + (\frac{\nu}{\pi})^{1/2}\frac{\Gamma((\nu-1)/2)}{\Gamma(\nu/2)}\delta$ and $Var(X) = (\sigma^2 + \delta^2)\frac{\nu}{\nu-2} - \frac{\nu}{\pi}\left[\frac{\Gamma((\nu-1)/2)}{\Gamma(\nu/2)}\right]^2\delta^2$, respectively. The parameter δ characterizes the skewness of the distribution. It is obvious that when δ goes to 0, the skew-t distribution degenerates to the usual symmetric Student t-distribution. The skew-t distribution proposed by Azzalini and Capitanio (2003) and Sahu et al. (2003) has different forms in multivariate case. But they are identical in the univariate case subject to a parameter transformation. Denote the form of Azzalini and Capitanio by $AST_\nu(\mu, s, \lambda)$. The two parameter sets have the following relationship: $s^2 = \sigma^2 + \delta^2$, $\lambda = \delta/\sigma$. The density of $AST_\nu(\mu, s, \lambda)$ is implemented in R package sn as $dst(x, location = \mu, scale = s, shape = \lambda, df = \nu)$. For convenience, we will denote the skew-t random effects model parameter by $\theta = (\mu, \lambda, \nu, \sigma_b, \sigma_e)$ in that order, where the skew-t distribution parameters are in the sense of Azzalini and Capitanio's AST; see Figure 3.7 for the density plot. However, Sahu et al.'s definition has the advantage of representing the skew-t distribution as a hierarchical way and thus is convenient for Bayesian parameter estimation as shown below.

According to Prentice (1974) and Lawless (1980), the log-gamma distribution was widely used in survival data analysis. However, the use of log-gamma distribution in general random effects model or linear mixed effects model was rarely seen in the literature. Recently, Zhang et al. (2008) proposed a non-normal linear mixed model where the random coefficients are assumed to be log-gamma distribution. The log-gamma distribution is left skewed, therefore, $-b_i$ is assumed to be log-gamma distributed. The density of log-gamma distribution can be written as

$$f(x|\alpha, \beta) = \frac{1}{\beta\Gamma(\alpha)}\exp\left(\alpha x/\beta - e^{x/\beta}\right)$$
(3.16)

where α is the shape parameter and β is the scale parameter. The mean and variance of log-gamma random variable are $\psi(\alpha)\beta$ and $\psi_1(\alpha)\beta^2$, where $\psi(\cdot)$ and $\psi_1(\cdot)$ are the digamma and trigamma function, respectively. As pointed out by Zhang et al. (2008), when the shape parameter α goes to infinity, the log-gamma distribution approaches the normal distribution. It is in this sense that the log-gamma distribution represents a broader class of distributions

Density Plot of Skew–t Distributions

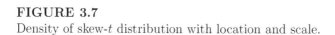

FIGURE 3.7

Density of skew-*t* distribution with location and scale.

which includes the normal distribution as a special case. Figure 3.8 is the density plot of log-gamma distribution with various parameters. Denote $\theta = (\mu, \alpha, \beta, \sigma_e)$, the marginal mean and variance of Y_{ij} in model (3.14) are $\mu - \psi(\alpha)\beta$ and $\psi_1(\alpha)\beta^2 + \sigma_e^2$, respectively. Because $-b_i$ follows the log-gamma distribution, there is a negative sign in the marginal mean as expected.

Computationally, Bayesian method can be used for parameter estimation mainly due to the convenience and flexibility of computational implementation thanks to the Bayesian computational tool `OpenBUGS` and its wrapper package in R called `BRugs`.

Following Jara et al. (2008), the skew-*t* random effects model can be hier-

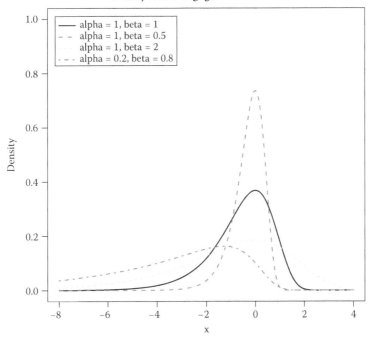

FIGURE 3.8
Density of log-gamma distribution with location and scale.

archically formulated as follows:

$$Y_{ij}|b_i \sim N(\mu + b_i, \sigma_e^2)$$
$$b_i|\gamma_i, \omega_i \sim N(\delta\gamma_i, \sigma_b^2/\omega_i)$$
$$\gamma_i \sim N(0, 1/\omega_i)I(\gamma_i > 0)$$
$$\omega_i \sim Gamma(\nu/2, \nu/2)$$

where γ_i and ω_i are augmented random variables used to generate skew-t random variable b_i. As pointed out by Jara et al. (2008), the location parameter of the above model is not identifiable. It is then necessary to reparameterize it as $\mu + (\frac{\nu}{\pi})^{1/2}\frac{\Gamma((\nu-1)/2)}{\Gamma(\nu/2)}\delta$ so that the random effect b_i has mean of 0.

The Bayesian computation method Markov chain Monte Carlo (MCMC) can be applied to obtain the posterior distribution. For Bayesian estimation, prior distribution is needed as part of model specification. Here, we will use vague priors for all the unknown parameters. Specifically, the priors for the parameters are assumed to be mutually independent and specified as follows:

$$\mu \sim N(0, 100)$$
$$1/\sigma_b^2 \sim Gamma(0.01, 0.01)$$
$$1/\sigma_e^2 \sim Gamma(0.01, 0.01)$$
$$\delta \sim N(0, 100)$$
$$\nu \sim Exp(0.1)I(\nu > 3)$$

The Bayesian computation of the log-gamma random effects model is straightforward given the following priors for its parameters:

$$\mu \sim N(0, 100)$$
$$\alpha \sim Gamma(0.01, 0.01)$$
$$1/\beta \sim Gamma(0.01, 0.01)$$

The posterior distributions can then be obtained through MCMC sampling method. The parameter estimations are determined as the median of their respective posterior distributions. After obtaining all the parameter estimations, which is denoted as $\hat{\theta}$, the cut point can be computed numerically. Denote the cut point as the pth quantile of the marginal distribution of Y, the cut point Q can then be estimated by solving the following equation numerically:

$$\int_{-\infty}^{Q} \int_{-\infty}^{\infty} \phi(y|b, \hat{\theta}) f(b|\hat{\theta}) db dy = p \qquad (3.17)$$

where $f(\cdot|\hat{\theta})$ is either the log-gamma density or skew-t density function with the estimated parameters; $\phi(\cdot|b, \hat{\theta})$ is the normal density function with mean $\hat{\mu} + b$ and variance $\hat{\sigma}_e^2$, conditioning on b.

To assess the performance of the proposed models, the cut point estimates are compared from computer simulations based on data generated from different underlying models. The simulated data are then fitted with normal, skew-t and log-gamma random effects models. The numbers of samples considered are 25, 50, 100 and the number of runs is 4. For each of these three combinations, 200 simulations are conducted. Parameter estimates are based on 5,000 MCMC samples after discarding 10,000 burn-in samples. The false positive rate is set to be 5%. For each simulated data, the cut point is estimated as the 95% quantile of the marginal distribution of each hypothesized model with unknown parameter replaced by its Bayesian estimate. For non-parametric method, the 95th quantile is calculated. Since quantiles are not directly comparable among different parameter settings, the empirical false positive rate under true model is also calculated. The mean and standard deviation of the cut point and its corresponding false positive rate under 200 simulations are reported. Simulation convergence is monitored by Heidelberger and Welch's (Heidelberger and Welch (1983)) convergence diagnostic.

For data generated from normal random effects model, the true parameter was set to be: (a) $\theta = (-0.1, 0.2, 0.05)$ and the true cut point was 0.239. As shown in Table 3.4, the skew-t random effects model always underestimates the cut point, consequently inflates the false positive rate by more than 1.2%. The log-gamma random effects model, on the other hand, always over-estimates the cut point, which deflates the false positive rate by more than 1.5%. Although the non-parametric estimation is expected to be unbiased, the method tends to under-estimate the cut point empirically when the number of samples is not large. In general, the non-parametric method is less efficient, as can be seen from the inflated standard deviation compared to its parametric counterpart. When the number of samples is small ($I = 25$), none of the models except the underlying one gives satisfactory results.

Two scenarios were considered for the underlying skew-t model: (b1) $\theta = (-1, 3, 5, 0.5, 0.1)$ and (b2) $\theta = (-1, 5, 8, 0.6, 0.1)$. These two scenarios represent different combinations of skewness and heaviness of the tail. The results were reported in Table 3.5 and 3.6, respectively. The results from these two scenarios show a similar pattern. The true cut points are 0.298 and 0.396, respectively. The Bayesian estimation of skew-t model results in downwards biased estimates as the sample size increases. This is mainly due to the less accurate estimate of the degree of freedom when the number of samples is not large enough. The bias becomes less severe when the sample size is getting larger, which implies that a large sample size is required to obtain nearly unbiased estimation. In terms of false positive rate, the skew-t model would inflate the false positive rate by at least 1% when the sample size is not large ($I = 25$ or 50). The normal model tends to inflate the false positive rate by a range from 1.4% to 3.1%. The log-gamma model also tends to under-estimate the cut points, but the deviation of false positive rate is within 1.2% when the number of samples is not small ($I = 50$ or 100). The non-parametric method gives more accurate estimation of the cut points than skew-t model itself, but is slightly less efficient as can be seen from the higher variability.

When the data are simulated from log-gamma model, the parameters are set to be (c1) $\theta = (0, 0.5, 0.1, 0.1)$ or (c2) $\theta = (0.1, 0.2, 0.05, 0.1)$. The true cut points are 0.648 and 0.890, respectively. As shown in Table 3.7 and 3.8, the normal and skew-t models would under-estimate the cut point and inflate false positive rate accordingly. On average, they will inflate the false positive rate by 2 percent. The non-parametric methods gives similar results to those from log-gamma estimations.

The simulation results were summarized as follows:

1) When the data are from normal random effects model, the skew-t model tends to under-estimate the cut point and inflate the false positive rate greatly; the log-gamma model will over-estimate the cut point and deflate the false positive rate significantly.

2) When the data are generated from skew-t model, all the methods under-estimate the cut points with inflated false positive rates. For the skew-t model itself, when the number of samples is small, the bias of false positive rate

TABLE 3.4

Comparison of cut point estimation (standard deviation in parentheses) from different models when the underlying model is normal (scenario a)

I	Normal		Skew-t		Log-Gamma		NP[a]	
	CP[b]	FR	CP	FR	CP	FR	CP	FR
25	0.241	0.055	0.217	0.069	0.319	0.029	0.226	0.068
	(0.057)	(0.030)	(0.059)	(0.034)	(0.088)	(0.036)	(0.074)	(0.042)
50	0.235	0.055	0.213	0.069	0.297	0.031	0.228	0.061
	(0.041)	(0.023)	(0.044)	(0.022)	(0.051)	(0.024)	(0.052)	(0.032)
100	0.240	0.051	0.221	0.062	0.301	0.028	0.235	0.055
	(0.029)	(0.015)	(0.040)	(0.021)	(0.035)	(0.021)	(0.037)	(0.020)

[a] NP: Non-Parametric Method.
[b] CP: Cut Point; FR: False Positive Rate.

estimate is quite significant and relatively large number of samples is suggested in practice to maintain a targeted false positive rate.

3) When the data are assumed to be from the log-gamma model, the normal and skew-*t* models tend to over-estimate the false positive rates dramatically.

4) The non-parametric method provides comparable but slightly less efficient cut point estimates to those from true parametric models. However, the parametric method has more to offer, such as magnitude and distribution of between-donor random effects.

The skew-*t* distribution appears to be less sensitive to outlying data values while taking the asymmetry and heavy tail into account; and thus has the advantage over the traditional robust method such as that based on median and MAD. Furthermore, the non-normal random effect model gives additional information regarding the distribution (and variability) of donors.

The impact of mis-specification of random effects may vary and need careful investigation. McCulloch and Neuhaus (2011) provided some results regarding parameter estimation and prediction but not on quantiles. Our simulation study showed that model mis-specification has large effect on the cut point estimation and the resulting false positive rate.

A real dataset from immunogenicity validation studies for detection of the ADAs against a monoclonal antibody therapeutic was reported by Zhang et al. (2015). The immunogenicity assay employed an electrochemi-luminescence (ECL) based format on Meso Scale Discovery (MSD) platform (Gaithersburg, MD). Aliquots of the antibody drug were labeled with biotin and ruthenium complex following procedures recommended by the manufacturer. Serum samples were diluted and incubated overnight with an equimolar mixture of the two labeled forms of the drug (ruthenylated and biotinylated). Under these conditions ADA molecules formed a bridge by binding simultaneously to both labeled forms of the drug. The reaction mixture was transferred to a pre-blocked streptavidin-coated plate for capture of ADA-drug complexes

TABLE 3.5
Comparison of cut point estimation(standard deviation in parentheses) from different models when the underlying model is skew-t (scenario b1)

	Normal		Skew-t		Log-Gamma		Nonparametric	
I	CP	FR	CP	FR	CP	FR	CP	FR
25	0.166	0.081	0.188	0.079	0.237	0.067	0.219	0.076
	(0.238)	(0.040)	(0.250)	(0.046)	(0.225)	(0.035)	(0.291)	(0.046)
50	0.210	0.069	0.250	0.063	0.261	0.060	0.290	0.061
	(0.194)	(0.029)	(0.195)	(0.030)	(0.173)	(0.024)	(0.255)	(0.032)
100	0.226	0.064	0.284	0.055	0.276	0.055	0.306	0.053
	(0.154)	(0.020)	(0.134)	(0.017)	(0.124)	(0.016)	(0.156)	(0.019)

TABLE 3.6
Comparison of cut point estimation(standard deviation in parentheses) from different models when the underlying model is skew-t (scenario b2)

	Normal		Skew-t		Log-Gamma		Nonparametric	
I	CP	FR	CP	FR	CP	FR	CP	FR
25	0.273	0.079	0.327	0.071	0.354	0.065	0.361	0.069
	(0.228)	(0.041)	(0.236)	(0.044)	(0.225)	(0.037)	(0.292)	(0.046)
50	0.263	0.076	0.350	0.062	0.342	0.062	0.374	0.061
	(0.158)	(0.030)	(0.172)	(0.027)	(0.161)	(0.026)	(0.224)	(0.032)
100	0.270	0.071	0.371	0.056	0.341	0.060	0.372	0.056
	(0.107)	(0.019)	(0.113)	(0.017)	(0.113)	(0.017)	(0.156)	(0.022)

TABLE 3.7
Comparison of cut point estimation(standard deviation in parentheses) from different models when the underlying model is log-gamma (scenario c1)

	Normal		Skew-t		Log-Gamma		Nonparametric	
I	CP	FR	CP	FR	CP	FR	CP	FR
25	0.592	0.074	0.600	0.074	0.807	0.054	0.631	0.066
	(0.095)	(0.036)	(0.085)	(0.040)	(0.134)	(0.033)	(0.126)	(0.042)
50	0.587	0.073	0.603	0.068	0.647	0.057	0.639	0.069
	(0.082)	(0.027)	(0.089)	(0.027)	(0.147)	(0.024)	(0.121)	(0.029)
100	0.592	0.068	0.619	0.060	0.651	0.053	0.641	0.055
	(0.056)	(0.018)	(0.058)	(0.017)	(0.098)	(0.017)	(0.072)	(0.018)

TABLE 3.8

Comparison of cut point estimation(standard deviation in parentheses) from different models when the underlying model is log-gamma (scenario c2)

I	Normal		Skew-t		Log-Gamma		Nonparametric	
	CP	FR	CP	FR	CP	FR	CP	FR
25	0.814	0.078	0.823	0.077	1.006	0.062	0.879	0.068
	(0.142)	(0.041)	(0.149)	(0.044)	(0.836)	(0.038)	(0.195)	(0.046)
50	0.803	0.077	0.825	0.071	0.867	0.061	0.874	0.061
	(0.102)	(0.028)	(0.108)	(0.028)	(0.133)	(0.025)	(0.139)	(0.031)
100	0.811	0.072	0.836	0.065	0.870	0.057	0.886	0.055
	(0.076)	(0.021)	(0.074)	(0.019)	(0.079)	(0.018)	(0.100)	(0.022)

by means of binding of the biotinylated drug to streptavidin. After one hour incubation followed by a wash step required to remove excessive reagents, the assay plate was treated with MSD Read Buffer and read immediately on MSD Sector Imager 6000. Screening and confirmatory evaluations were performed on the same assay plate. Confirmatory wells were treated the same as the screening assay wells, except for the presence of excess unlabeled drug. The ECL counts of all the plate wells were recorded.

Fifty samples were tested in four runs with each run using four plates. Individual samples were tested in duplicated wells on each plate and the mean ECL signal was calculated. Pooled negative samples from 8 wells on each plate served as negative control. The screening assay results (signal to background or SB) for each sample was obtained by dividing the mean ECL signal of the duplicate wells by the mean ECL response of negative control from the same plate. Log transformation on SB was taken before statistical analysis. One donor had an average value greater than 4.0 (on natural log scale) across the four runs. This donor could be a biological outlier and it was decided to remove this donor before the analysis. Later on, that donor was added back to check the robustness of the skew-t model. The upper panel of Figure 3.9 showed the empirical density plot of the 196 SB values on the natural log scale. Without taking into account the donor heterogeneity, the empirical distribution was compared with the fitted skew-t distribution as well as normal and log-gamma distributions. The skew-t model appeared to be a good candidate. We then fitted a skew-t random effects model to the data. As a comparison, the other models were also fitted to the data. The parameter estimate for the skew-t random effects model was $\theta = (-0.075, 1.933, 4.088, 0.127, 0.073)$ using the same method as in the simulation study. The cut point estimates from the various models were listed in the first row of Table 3.9. Including all the data, the parameter estimate was $\theta = (-0.078, 1.908, 3.278, 0.125, 0.072)$. Except for the degree of freedom, the other parameter estimates were very close to each other. The cut point estimates are listed in the second row of Table 3.9. It can be seen that the skew-t model gave a relative robust estimate of the

TABLE 3.9
Comparison of cut point estimation from different random effects models

Normal	Skew-t	Log-Gamma	Non-Parametric
0.387	0.299	0.314	0.306
1.168	0.321	0.627	0.407

cut point as compared to other models as well as the non-parametric method; the latter is sensitive to outliers, however.

Formal model goodness of fit and diagnostics remain to be a challenging problem for non-normal random effects model. Here we use informal graphical display to show the goodness of fit. As shown in the bottom of Figure 3.9, the random effects prediction obtained from the normal random effects model was plotted against the densities of all the fitted random effects models. The skew-t model showed remarkably better fit than the normal distribution because it can not only capture the skewness but also the heavy tail. The log-gamma model also fitted the data very well. Although the deviance information criteria (Spiegelhalter et al. (2002)) showed that log-gamma random effects model was better than the skew-t model, the skew-t model may be preferred due to its robustness.

3.3.3   Comparison of Cut Point Methods

3.3.3.1   Data Including Positive Donors

Jaki et al. (2011) considered various situations where true positive and true negative are mixed together and compared the performance of different cut point determination methods. Such effort is worthwhile in certain circumstances, for example, when a significant portion of pre-existing antibodies is known to exist in the data. In general, the performance of a cut point to correctly classify donors as positive or negative depends on the separation of the distributions between positive and negative donors. For a given dataset consisting of both positive and negative donors, there is always a trade-off of the cut point. As shown in Figure 3.10, increasing cut point will decrease the false positive rate α while inflating the false negative rate β. It is known that false positive classification is the sponsor's risk while false negative classification is the patients' risk. Therefore, it is desirable to have more false positives than more false negatives. Jaki et al. (2011) conducted a comprehensive simulation study to compare various cut point methods given the mixed data with both true negatives and true positives. The results indicate that robust method perform best for ensuring low false negative rate and high proportion of true positive classifications. This is expected as the robust method gives conservative cut point values compared to other methods. The mixture model method

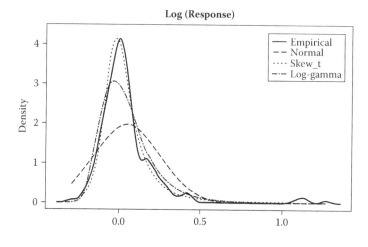

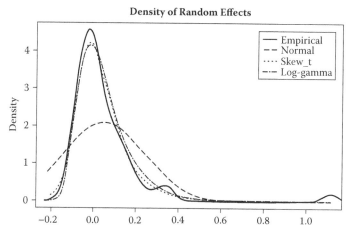

FIGURE 3.9

Comparison of empirical distribution with fitted distributions for marginal response and estimated random effects.

proposed by Jaki et al. (2011) also performs well and is particularly useful for data including true positives.

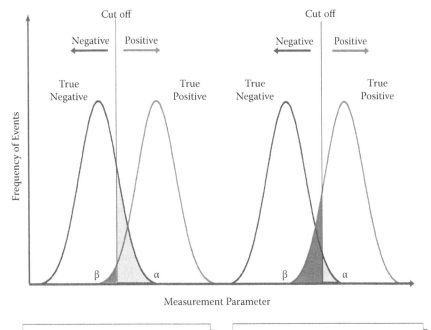

FIGURE 3.10
The impact of cut point on data where positive and negative donors are mixed together. Courtesy of Dr. Robert Kubiak.

3.3.3.2 Prediction Interval and Tolerance Interval

The quantile estimator `mean` $+ 1.645 * sqrt($`total variability`$)$ under a normality assumption as a cut point is in fact not an unbiased estimator of the true quantile and thus gives rise to slight deviation from 5% false positive rate when applied to future data with the same normal distribution. Hoffman and Berger (2011) compared different cut point estimators including non-parametric quantile, parametric quantile, robust method, and upper prediction bound assuming the underlying model is a normal random effect model. To maintain 5% false positive rate, they recommended the prediction limit over the quantile. A prediction limit or prediction interval is an estimate of a limit/interval in which a future data point (y_f) with the same population distribution will fall with a certain probability. For example, the prediction upper limit for normal distribution is simply $\bar{y}_n + t_{1-\alpha,n-1}s_n\sqrt{1+1/n}$. To construct such prediction interval/limit, recognize that

$$\frac{y_f - \bar{y}_n}{\sqrt{1+1/n}s_n} \sim t(n-1). \tag{3.18}$$

For random effect models such as the following two-way random effect model:

$$y_{ij} = \mu + \alpha_i + \beta_j + \epsilon_{ij}, \tag{3.19}$$

It is not difficult to derive that $y_f - \overline{y}$ is normally distributed with mean 0 and variance $\sigma_{y_f}^2 + \sigma_{\overline{y}}^2$, where $\sigma_{y_f}^2$ and $\sigma_{\overline{y}}^2$ are the variance of y_f and $\overline{y}$, respectively, with y_f following the above two-way random effect model. Therefore, the $1 - \alpha$ upper prediction limit can be found to be $\overline{y} + t_{1-\alpha,df}\sqrt{\hat{\sigma}_{y_f}^2 + \hat{\sigma}_{\overline{y}}^2}$, where $t_{1-\alpha,df}$ is the $100(1 - \alpha)$-th lower quantile of t-distribution with degree-of-freedom df; the degree of freedom df can be estimated via Satterthwaite (1946) approximation. Hoffman and Berger (2011) conducted simulation to compare the false positive rates for various cut point methods. Their simulation studies show that the upper prediction bound best maintains the targeted false positive rate on average while the variation around the targeted false positive rate is minimal among the methods mentioned above. The parametric quantile fails to maintain the targeted false positive rate when the sample size is not large enough. For these reasons, Hoffman and Berger (2011) recommended using the prediction limit for cut point determination.

While the upper prediction limit maintains targeted false positive rate in the average sense, there is still 50% chance that it will give rise to a false positive rate being less than the targeted false positive rate in a single study. The deviation to the targeted false positive rate can sometimes be immense. Hoffman and Berger (2011) argued that a confidence-level cut point approach may be utilized to ensure that the chance of being less than the targeted false positive rate is as small as, say, 5%. This leads to the concept of tolerance limit or tolerance bound. The tolerance limit is such that with some confidence level, a specified proportion of population samples will be within the bound. Equivalently, the confidence bound of the quantile is pursued, instead of the quantile itself. The one-sided tolerance limit is nothing but the one-sided confidence bound for the unknown quantile of interest. Consider independently and identically distributed (IID) data $X_1, X_2, , X_n$ with underlying distribution $F(\theta)$ whose $100(1 - \alpha)$th quantile is q or $q(1 - \alpha)$. Then, the $100(1 - \beta)$ level one-sided confidence limit, or equivalently, the $100(1 - \beta)$ level p-content lower tolerance limit is

$$Pr[Pr(X > Q(X_1, , X_n)) \geq p] = 1 - \beta \tag{3.20}$$

which can be re-written as $Pr(Q(X1, , X_n) \leq q(p)) = 1 - \beta$, or $P(FPR \geq \alpha) = 1 - \beta$. The former indicates that the lower tolerance limit is *de facto* confidence limit for the true cut point $q(1 - \alpha)$, while the latter guarantees the false positive rate has $100(1-\beta)\%$ confidence of being greater than the targeted false positive rate α. Shen et al. (2015) compared the quantile estimator with the lower tolerance limit under IID normal assumption. As expected, the quantile estimator has mean false positive rate of 5% in their simulation study while the tolerance limit has about 95% confidence of having greater than 5% false positive rate. When considering the data from multiple runs, they are no longer

IID, but correlated. The tolerance limit for random effect models can be used for "confidence-level" cut point. Krishnamoorthy and Mathew (2009) reviewed different approaches to constructing tolerance bound for various models such as one-way and two-way random effect models. Hoffman (2010) proposed a simple method for multi-way random effects model.

3.3.3.3 Confirmatory Cut Point

Alternative methods for confirmatory cut point determination were proposed. Neyer et al. (2006) proposed to use the t-test to declare positivity. Specifically, data from multiple runs are available before and after label-free excess drug in the confirmatory assay for each donor. The donor is declared to be positive if the p-value of the t-test is less than 0.01 for a false positive of 1%. Separately, Jaki et al. (2014) used the difference between the data before and after label-free excess drug. In the simulation study conducted by Jaki et al. (2014) assuming data including true positives, they found that both the method of difference and t-test are better than the inhibition method introduced in Section 3.2.

Wakshull and Coleman (2011) argued that the confirmatory assay data should be orthogonal to the screening assay data in order to provide maximal information to eliminate false positives from screening assay. Confirmatory assay should be optimized in light of this objective. However, Kubiak et al. (2013) found through their experience that the screening assay data and confirmatory assay data often demonstrated rather high correlation, and thus question the usefulness of the confirmatory assay. While the findings are interesting, evaluation of the screening data and confirmatory data together theoretically is rather challenging.

As can be seen from the above discussion, there are many questions still remain unanswered for the tiered approach to immunogenicity assay. Continuous efforts from scientists and statisticians are still needed for more research in this area.

4

Clinical Immunogenicity Assessment

CONTENTS

4.1 Introduction

In the past few decades, an increasing number of patients are benefiting from treatment with newly developed biologics. Among them, monoclonal antibodies (mAbs), representing a large class of biologics that are highly specific to their targets, have been successful in treating various cancers and autoimmune diseases. However, like other biologics, most protein therapeutics including mAbs elicit a certain level of undesirable ADA responses which may negatively impact product efficacy and/or safety. There have been many achievements of improving tolerability and reducing the immunogenicity of mAbs. Humanized mAbs, which contain replacement of mouse constant regions by human sequences, are less immunogenic than chimeric or murine mAbs. However, humanized and even fully human sequence-derived mAbs may still carry immunological risk. As a requirement of biologics license application (BLA) and Marketing Authorization Application (MAA), the potential impact of the ADA responses on overall clinical efficacy and safety should be characterized and clearly understood as emphasized in Chapter 1. The requirements include validated immunogenicity assays for screening and identifying patients with positive ADA responses and assessment of the ADA impact on clinical benefit and risk.

The first step of assessing the clinical risk of immunogenicity is the development of reliable immunogenicity assays that can detect, quantify and characterize the ADA responses accurately. There are several major challenges in the assessment of the immunogenic potential of biologics. As summarized by Wolbink et al. (2009), an ADA response has a diverse range from low-affinity IgM antibodies to high-affinity IgG antibodies. There is no available assay that can universally detect all different forms of antibodies. In addition, the immunogenicity assay may have interference with the presence of the drug. Therefore, analytical methods used for testing immunogenicity should be properly developed, optimized and validated before the method is used in non-clinical and clinical testings (Shankar et al. (2008)). In Chapters 2 and 3, various issues in ADA assay development and validation have been discussed extensively.

Many bioanalytical methods are available to predict the immunogenicity of a biologic based on animal models or *in silico*. But the use of animal models needs critical evaluation. Because of species differences, the predictive value of animal models for the potential of ADA formation in human is limited, and mechanistic studies may be restricted (ICH S6, Brinks et al. (2011)). For example, 100% of cynomolgus monkeys treated with Humira, a recombinant human mAb for treating arthritis, Crohn's disease, and other autoimmune diseases, developed ADA, but the immunogenicity rate in clinical trials was only 12% (Ponce et al. (2009)). Therefore, the impact of immunogenicity on efficacy and safety can only be ultimately evaluated using data from clinical trials or post-marketing surveillance. A thorough understanding of the incidence, kinetics, duration and magnitude of the ADA responses along with the neutralizing ability is required to assess the clinical impact of a given biologics. In the end, an immunogenicity risk assessment program should be aimed to mitigate the risk of clinical immunogenicity and to enhance the clinical management of patients.

Shankar et al. (2014) gave some commonly-used definitions and terminologies for the description of immunogenicity and provided guidance on the types of information that is needed to evaluate the clinical risk of immunogenicity. In this chapter, we provide a comprehensive review of the statistical methods that can be used to assess the impact of ADA in clinical studies. Various statistical methods are presented and applied to data from a hypothetical clinical trial that investigates the efficacy and safety of a novel mAb for the treatment of rheumatoid arthritis (RA). Section 4.2 contains general information about RA including symptoms, causes, and treatment. This section also includes a description of the hypothetical clinical trial, and clinical ADA assay methods. In the subsequent sections, statistical approaches with focus on the evaluation of clinical immunogenicity data are presented. We introduce some basic terminologies, e.g., incidence and prevalence, for the description of clinical immunogenicity. We describe the statistical methods for calculating and comparing the ADA incidence rates between the control and treatment groups. Using the status of ADA responses as the risk factor, we discuss a wide range of statistical techniques for examining the effect of ADA on efficacy and safety. Depending on the type of endpoints, relevant statistical methods like generalized linear models, survival analysis, longitudinal data analysis, and generalized additive models are presented and applied to the hypothetical clinical trial data. We also discuss some special topics, for example survival analysis with recurrent events, interval-censoring, and multiplicity adjustment in the adverse event (AE) analysis. In addition to existence of ADA responses, ADA titer is another important response that measures the magnitude of ADA in patient samples. Because of the special characteristics of ADA titer, some special statistical methods like log-transformation and zero-inflated models are considered.

4.2 Monoclonal Antibodies for the Treatment of Rheumatoid Arthritis (RA)

RA is a serious autoimmune disease that typically affects linings of the small joints in hands and feet. RA causes a painful swelling that can eventually result in bone erosion and joint deformity. In addition to causing joint problems, complications from RA include other body parts such as the skin, eyes, lungs, and blood vessels. Because some diseases, such as scleroderma and lupus, have symptoms similar to RA, a differential diagnosis is required. The onset time of RA is usually after age 40, although the symptoms can appear at any age. Gender is a significant risk factor and the disorder is much more prevalent among women than men. Worldwide, about 0.13% men and 0.35% women suffer from RA (Cross et al. (2014)). In the United States, nearly three times as many women have the disease as men (http://www.arthritis.org/arthritis-facts/disease-center/rheumatoid-arthritis.php). Currently, there is no cure for RA and the available treatments can only manage the symptoms and slow the progression of joint damage (Agarwal (2011)).

Treatment of RA with synthetic disease-modifying anti-rheumatoid drugs (DMARDs), such as methotrexate, leflunomide and sufasalazine, has led to remarkable improvement in clinical symptoms and slower joint damage (Fan and Leong (2007); Agarwal (2011); Bossaller and Rothe (2013)). Although conventional DMARDs are considered as the standard of care for most patients, a significant number of patients do not have adequate responses to one or more DMARDs (Hider et al. (2005)). With recent advances in the understanding of the pathogenesis of RA, novel cellular and molecular therapeutic targets, such as TNFα and interleukin-6 (IL-6), have been identified. With these advances, an increasing number of biologics, including mAbs, with various mechanisms of action (MoA) have been developed and approved for the treatment of RA (Bossaller and Rothe (2013)).

The majority of mAbs approved for the treatment of RA target tumor necrosis factor TNFα (Agarwal (2011)), which contributes to the inflammation in affected joints. Used alone or in combination with the DMARDs, mAbs have been successful in relieving symptoms in patients with moderate to severe RA. Additionally, biologics have been shown to slow the progression of RA when all the other treatments have failed to do so. By combining DMARDs and biologics, the management of RA has been transformed over the last two decades. Now, emerging biological agents offer RA patients great hope of prolonged or even permanent remission.

Despite the success of biologics in reducing clinical symptoms of RA patients, acute and chronic AEs occur (Rubbert-Roth (2012)). A common acute but potentially fatal side effect is the infusion reactions due to the "cytokine storm," a massive release of cytokines like IL-2, IL-6 and TNFα. The cytokine release syndrome typically appears shortly after the administration of the drug and may last for several hours. The use of biologics may also increase the risk of infections. RA patients should be screened annually for tuberculosis and receive pneumococcal, influenza and hepatitis B vaccinations (Agarwal (2011)). Another common side effect is the formation of ADAs, which may neutralize the drug activity and lead to the loss of therapeutic efficacy or accelerated drug clearance, shortening the length of its effect.

4.2.1 Hypothetical Clinical Trial of an mAb Drug for RA

We consider a hypothetical clinical trial that evaluates the efficacy and safety of an mAb as a novel treatment for RA. In the randomized, double-blinded, placebo-controlled clinical trial, 600 patients with moderate to severe RA were randomly assigned to receive injections of an experimental mAb (Drug $\mathcal{X}$) or placebo subcutaneously. To examine the dose–response relationship, patients were randomized into four treatment groups (150 patients/group) to receive either placebo, or one of the three dose levels (20mg, 40mg, and 80mg). Drug $\mathcal{X}$ was administered every four weeks on Weeks 0 (day 1), 4 and 8 for the first 3 doses and thereafter every 8 weeks on weeks 16, 24, 32, 40, 48, and 56 for the next 6 doses. The patients were then followed during the treatment to assess the efficacy and safety. ADA levels were evaluated prior to the first dose and at pre-defined intervals through the end of the study (56 weeks).

The primary endpoint of the study was RA remission. According to the criteria of the American College of Rheumatology (ACR) (Makinen et al. (2006)), RA remission is defined as "five or more of the following requirements be fulfilled for at least two consecutive months:"

(1) Duration of morning stiffness not exceeding 15 minutes

(2) No fatigue

(3) No joint pain by history

(4) No joint tenderness or pain in motion

(5) No soft tissue swelling in joints or tendon sheaths

(6) Erythrocyte sedimentation rate by Westergren method: $< 30 \text{ mm/h}$ for women or 20 mm/h for men.

The secondary endpoint was the modified Disease Activity Score using 28 joint count (DAS28), which is a validated index of RA disease activity (Mäkinen et al. (2005)). DAS28 is a composite measure based on four disease scores: 28 tender joint count (TJC28), swollen joint count (SJC) counts, erythrocyte sedimentation rate (ESR), and patient's global health (GH). The DAS28 index was calculated using the formula: $0.56 \times \sqrt{\text{TJC28}} + 0.28 \times \sqrt{\text{SJC28}} + 0.70 \times \sqrt{\log(\text{ESR})} + 0.014 \times \text{GH}$. In the trial, DAS28 scores were measured at weeks 0, 4, 8, 16, 24, 32, 40, 48, and 56 for each patient. AEs were recorded according to the Medical Dictionary for Regulatory Activities (MedRA) system organ class (Brown et al. (1999)). In the case of treatment withdrawal, the date and reasons for the withdrawal were recorded by the clinical investigators. Withdrawal due to treatment-related AEs was defined as a failure due to adverse drug reaction.

4.2.2 ADA Testing Protocol

Blood samples for ADA assessment were taken prior to drug administration on Day 1 and on all subsequent treatment visits. A tiered testing scheme for ADA responses to the mAb consisted of screening, confirmatory, and titering assays. The screening assay cut point and the confirmatory assay cut point were determined using the statistical method described in Chapter 3 based on validation samples. The validation sample data were obtained from 200 measurements of serum samples from 50 additional drug-naive disease subjects. Once the screening cut point and confirmatory cut point were determined from the validation data, samples for subjects in the clinical trial were first screened for the presence of ADA. Samples that measured at or above the screening cut point were considered potentially ADA positive to Drug $\mathcal{X}$ and were retested by the confirmatory assay. Samples were determined as ADA positive when the mAb caused the ADA response to a level greater than or equal to the confirmatory cut point, which was established using a 1% false positive rate. The ADA titer was determined subsequently. Titers were reported as the reciprocal of the highest dilution that produced a positive result. ADA status and titer were evaluated at Day 1 (week 0), and weeks 4, 16, 24, 32, 40, 48, and 56.

4.2.3 Analysis Diagram

Proper risk assessment of clinical immunogenicity considers both the probability and the magnitude of generating an immune response and its consequences on efficacy and safety. The analysis of clinical immunogenicity involves three primary components: treatment and dose regime X, clinical responses

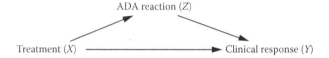

FIGURE 4.1
Relationship between treatment, immunogenicity and clinical efficacy.

Y and immunogenicity response Z. Figure 4.1 shows the relationship between the treatment, ADA reaction and clinical responses. Treatment with biologics (X) has the potential to induce ADA formation (Z), and ADA can potentially impact clinical efficacy (Y).

In this hypothetical model, the most relevant variable for treatment is dose level. However, clinical trials are often more complex and the effects of additional treatment variables such as administration route, dosing regime and inclusion of combination therapy arms may require evaluation for their effects on the development of ADA. ADA responses, e.g., prevalent and incident cases of ADA, ADA onset time and duration, magnitude of ADA responses measured by titers, may be heterogeneous,. The clinical responses can be efficacy measures, e.g., overall survival, disease-free survival (remission), longitudinal biomarkers and/or AEs. Given different characteristics of the ADA and clinical responses, a wide array of statistical techniques can be used to examine the relationships between X, Y and Z. In a broader sense, baseline variables and patient characteristics can be analyzed as covariates in a similar way as the treatment.

4.3 Statistical Analysis of ADA Status

Depending on the initiation and occurrence times, ADA responses can be classified into various types (Shankar et al. (2014)). Prevalent ADA response are present in the patient population within a short period of time or a specific time point prior to initial drug treatment. Incident ADAs, also known as treatment-emergent ADAs, are ADA responses that develop at some point after the initial treatment with the biologics (Shankar et al. (2014)). Incident ADAs also include patients who were ADA-positive prior to treatment that had increases, also known as boosts, in ADA response following treatment.

Regardless of the actual type of an ADA response, the status of an ADA response can be classified as positive or negative by immunogenicity testing.

Let $Y = I$(Positive ADA response) denote the binary random variable for ADA status with the indicator function $I(\cdot)$, where $Y = 1$ for a positive ADA response and $Y = 0$ for a negative ADA response. A Bernoulli distribution is often used for the binary random variable:

$$Y \sim \text{Bernoulli}(\pi), \qquad (4.1)$$

where π is the probability of a positive ADA response.

Suppose that there are n subjects in the study. Let Y_i be the binary ADA status for the ith subject. The total number of subjects with positive response is $S = \sum_i Y_i$. Then the number of ADA positive responses S is distributed as a binomial distribution with success probability π:

$$P(S = s) = \text{Binomial}(n, \pi) = \binom{n}{s} \pi^s (1 - \pi)^{n-s},$$

where $E(S) = n\pi$ and $V(S) = n\pi(1 - \pi)$. The unbiased estimate of π is $\hat{\pi} = s/n$, which is also the maximum likelihood estimate (MLE) . In this section, we will describe the statistical inference of ADA status. For a comprehensive review of the assessment of relative risk and categorical data analysis, see Lachin (2014) and Agresti (2014).

4.3.1   Confidence Intervals of ADA Response Rates

Asymptotically the estimate of ADA response rate $\hat{\pi}$ follows a normal distribution

$$\hat{\pi} \sim N\left(\pi, \frac{\pi(1 - \pi)}{n}\right).$$

The confidence interval (CI) of π is often constructed based on a logit transformation. Let $\theta = \log[\pi/(1 - \pi)]$, the asymptotic distribution of $\hat{\theta}$ (Durrett (2010)) is

$$\hat{\theta} = \log\left(\frac{\hat{\pi}}{1 - \hat{\pi}}\right) \sim N\left[\log\left(\frac{\pi}{1 - \pi}\right), \frac{1}{n\pi(1 - \pi)}\right].$$

The symmetric $(1 - \alpha)$ CI for θ is

$$(\hat{\theta}_L, \hat{\theta}_U) = \hat{\theta} \pm Z_{1-\alpha/2}\sqrt{\frac{1}{n\hat{\pi}(1 - \hat{\pi})}},$$

where $Z_{1-\alpha}$ is the $(1 - \alpha)$ quantile of the standard normal distribution. The asymmetric confidence limits of π can be obtained by inverting the logit function,

$$(\hat{\pi}_L, \hat{\pi}_U) = \left(\frac{\exp(\hat{\theta}_L)}{1 + \exp(\hat{\theta}_L)}, \frac{\exp(\hat{\theta}_U)}{1 + \exp(\hat{\theta}_U)}\right).$$

The CIs of the ADA response probability π can also be constructed using other methods, e.g., the exact method, test-inverted method (Lachin (2014)). Besides the logit transformation, probit or complementary-log-log transformations are also used for proportions.

4.3.2 Comparison of ADA Response Rates

In addition to the CIs of ADA response rates within each treatment group, it is of interest to compare the ADA response rates across different groups. Let n_1 and n_2 denote the numbers of subjects for the two groups under comparison, and the numbers of positive ADA responses from the two groups are S_1 and S_2, respectively. The positive responses follow binomial distributions as $S_i \sim$ Binomial$(n_i, \pi_i), i = 1, 2$. Without loss of generality, we use the capital letter to denote the random variable and use the corresponding lower-case letter to denote the observed value of the random variable. For example, the observed number of ADA+ cases is s_i for group $i, i = 1, 2$. The resulting data of two-group comparison are usually summarized in a 2×2 table:

TABLE 4.1
The 2×2 table for ADA responses in two groups.

ADA status	Group 1	Group 2	
+	s_1	s_2	m_1
−	$n_1 - s_1$	$n_2 - s_2$	m_2
All	n_1	n_2	n

Measures of comparing the response rates between two subgroups include the risk ratio (RR) and odds ratio (OR). The RR is defined as RR $= \pi_2/\pi_1$, the ratio of the probabilities of positive ADA responses in the two groups; and the OR is defined as OR $= \frac{\pi_2/(1-\pi_2)}{\pi_1/(1-\pi_1)}$, the ratio of the odds of positive ADA responses in the two groups. Both the RR and the OR take positive value from $\mathbb{R}^+ = (0, \infty)$. When the ADA response rates from the two groups are equal, both measures of relative risk are 1.0.

Because the natural estimates of response probability are sample proportions $\hat{\pi}_1 = s_1/n_1$ and $\hat{\pi}_2 = s_2/n_2$, the estimates of RR and OR can be obtained by substituting the proportion estimates $\hat{\pi}_i$. Therefore,

$$\widehat{RR} = \hat{\pi}_2/\hat{\pi}_1 = \frac{s_2/n_2}{s_1/n_1},$$

$$\widehat{OR} = \frac{\hat{\pi}_2/(1 - \hat{\pi}_2)}{\hat{\pi}_1/(1 - \hat{\pi}_1)} = \frac{s_2(n_1 - s_1)}{s_1(n_2 - s_2)}.$$

To obtain a symmetric distribution of the RR and OR, one usually takes a logarithm transformation (Lachin (2014)). Asymptotically,

$$E[\log(\widehat{RR})] \quad = \quad \log(RR) = \log(\pi_2) - \log(\pi_1), \tag{4.2}$$

$$V[\log(\widehat{RR})] \quad = \quad \frac{1 - \pi_1}{n_1 \pi_1} + \frac{1 - \pi_2}{n_2 \pi_2} \tag{4.3}$$

The consistent estimate of (4.3) is

$$\hat{\sigma}^2_{\log RR} = \hat{V}[\log(\widehat{RR})] = \frac{1 - \hat{\pi}_1}{n_1 \hat{\pi}_1} + \frac{1 - \hat{\pi}_2}{n_2 \hat{\pi}_2} = \frac{1}{s_1} - \frac{1}{n_1} + \frac{1}{s_2} - \frac{1}{n_2}. \tag{4.4}$$

The large-sample $(1 - \alpha)$ CI of $\theta = \log(RR)$ is

$$(\hat{\theta}_L, \hat{\theta}_U) = \log\left(\frac{\hat{\pi}_2}{\hat{\pi}_1}\right) \pm Z_{1-\alpha/2}\hat{\sigma}_{\log RR} \tag{4.5}$$

The CI for the RR is then obtained as $(\widehat{RR}_L, \widehat{RR}_U) = (\exp(\hat{\theta}_L), \exp(\hat{\theta}_U))$.
Similarly, the asymptotic expectation and variance of $\log(OR)$ are

$$E[\log(\widehat{OR})] \quad = \quad \log(OR) = \log\left(\frac{\pi_2}{1 - \pi_2}\right) - \log\left(\frac{\pi_1}{1 - \pi_1}\right), \tag{4.6}$$

$$V[\log(\widehat{OR})] \quad = \quad \frac{1}{n_1 \pi_1 (1 - \pi_1)} + \frac{1}{n_2 \pi_2 (1 - \pi_2)}. \tag{4.7}$$

The variance of $\log(\widehat{OR})$ can be estimated as

$$\hat{\sigma}^2_{\log OR} = \hat{V}[\log(\widehat{OR})] = \frac{1}{n_1 \hat{\pi}_1 (1 - \hat{\pi}_1)} + \frac{1}{n_2 \hat{\pi}_2 (1 - \hat{\pi}_2)} \tag{4.8}$$

Likewise, the large-sample $(1 - \alpha)$ CI for $\theta = \log(OR)$ is

$$(\hat{\theta}_L, \hat{\theta}_U) = \log\left(\frac{\hat{\pi}_2/(1 - \hat{\pi}_2)}{\hat{\pi}_1/(1 - \hat{\pi}_1)}\right) \pm Z_{1-\alpha/2}\hat{\sigma}_{\log OR} \tag{4.9}$$

The CI for the OR is constructed as $(\widehat{OR}_L, \widehat{OR}_U) = (\exp(\hat{\theta}_L), \exp(\hat{\theta}_U))$.

4.3.3   Statistical Tests of ADA Response Rates

In addition to the large-sample distribution of the relative risks, one can further test the statistical significance of the difference of ADA response rates for the two groups. The hypotheses to be tested are the null hypothesis $H_0 : \pi_1 = \pi_2$ versus the alternative hypothesis $H_1 : \pi_1 \neq \pi_2$. Under the null hypothesis, the rates of positive ADA responses are the same for the two groups. For a large sample size, a variety of approaches can be used to perform the test, e.g., the chi-square test and Fisher's exact test. There are two types of likelihood specifications based on the sampling models for the population. First, one can assume that the observed ADA+ responses S_1 and S_2

in Table 4.1 come from two independent binomial distributions with sample sizes n_1 and n_2 from two different populations. The resulting function is an unconditional product-binomial likelihood

$$
\begin{aligned}
L_B(\pi_1, \pi_2) &= P(S_1 = s_1, S_2 = s_2) = P(S_1 = s_1 | n_1, \pi_1) P(S_2 = s_2 | n_2, \pi_2) \\
&= \binom{n_1}{s_1} \pi_1^{s_1} (1 - \pi_1)^{n_1 - s_1} \binom{n_2}{s_2} \pi_2^{s_2} (1 - \pi_2)^{n_2 - s_2}. \quad (4.10)
\end{aligned}
$$

The most commonly used test statistic is the Pearson chi-square X_P^2 for a general $R \times C$ contingency table with R rows and C columns. For a 2×2 table, the test statistic X_P^2 can calculated as

$$
X_P^2 = \frac{[s_1(n_2 - s_1) - s_2(n_1 - s_1)]^2 n}{n_1 n_2 m_1 m_2}. \quad (4.11)
$$

Under the null hypothesis, X_P^2 follows a chi-square distribution with one degrees of freedom (DF). Therefore, H_0 would be rejected when $X_P^2 \geq \chi^2_{1-\alpha}$, the $1 - \alpha$ percentile of the central χ^2 distribution.

The unconditional likelihood (4.10) can be expressed in terms of the total number of positive responses M_1 since $M_1 = S_1 + S_2$. Let $\theta = \frac{\pi_2/(1-\pi_2)}{\pi_1/(1-\pi_1)}$ be the OR. The probability of observing $(S_1 = s_1, S_2 = s_2)$ can be expressed as

$$
\begin{aligned}
P(S_1 = s_1, M_1 = m_1) &= P(S_1 = s_1, S_2 = m_1 - s_1) \\
&= \binom{n_1}{s_1} \binom{n_1}{m_1 - s_1} \theta^{s_2} (1 - \pi_2)^{n_2} \pi_1^{m_1} (1 - \pi_1)^{n_1 - m_1}.
\end{aligned}
$$

The conditional likelihood function, conditioning on total number of ADA+ cases M_1 being fixed, can be obtained as

$$
\begin{aligned}
L_C(\theta) &= \frac{P(S_1 = s_1, M_1 = m_1)}{P(M_1 = m_1)} \\
&= \frac{\binom{n_1}{s_1}\binom{n_2}{s_2}\theta^{s_2}}{\sum_{i=L}^{U} \binom{n_1}{i}\binom{n_2}{m_1 - i}\theta^{i}}, \quad (4.12)
\end{aligned}
$$

where $L = \max(0, m_1 - n_2)$ and $U = \min(m_1, n_1)$. The likelihood $L_C(\theta)$ is the conditional noncentral hypergeometric distribution with noncentrality parameter θ.

With the transformation $\theta = \frac{\pi_2/(1-\pi_2)}{\pi_1/(1-\pi_1)}$, the null hypothesis $H_0 : \pi_1 = \pi_2$ is equivalent to $H_0 : \theta = 1$. Then the condition likelihood function under the null hypothesis reduces to a central hypergeometric distribution

$$
L_C(\theta = 1) = \frac{\binom{n_1}{s_1}\binom{n_2}{s_2}}{\binom{n}{m_1}}. \quad (4.13)
$$

The resulting statistical test is called the Fisher's exact test (Fisher (1922)). The p-value of the Fisher's exact test can be obtained from SAS PROC FREQ and other statistical packages.

4.3.4   Dose–Response Model of ADA Response

The Fisher's exact test and the Pearson's χ^2 test can be used to compare the ADA response rates between two groups. However, such tests cannot be used to detect a dose–response relationship. When there are multiple treatment groups, particularly with increasing doses, it is often useful to assess whether the ADA response rates increase with dose. The dose–response data are usually organized in a $2 \times K$ table.

TABLE 4.2

The $2 \times K$ table of ADA dose–response data in multiple dose groups

	Dose d_1	Dose d_2	$\cdots$	Dose d_K
Number of ADA+ responses	s_1	s_2	$\cdots$	s_K
Number of subjects	n_1	n_2	$\cdots$	n_K

In Table 4.2, there are K dose groups with dose levels $d_1 < d_2 < \cdots < d_K$. The number of positive ADA response follows a Binomial distribution $S_i \sim$ Binomial(n_i, π_i) for dose group $d_i, i = 1, ..., K$. Usually, $d_1 = 0$ is the dose level for the placebo group. The Cochran–Armitage (CA) trend test (Cochran (1954b); Armitage (1955)) considers the following hypothesis of increasing trends:

$$H_0 : \pi_1 = \pi_2 = \cdots = \pi_K \tag{4.14}$$

versus

$$H_1 : \pi_1 \leq \pi_2 \leq \cdots \leq \pi_K \text{ with at least one unequal sign.} \tag{4.15}$$

Cochran (1954b) and Armitage (1955) considered a linear response probability model

$$\pi_i = \alpha + \beta d_i, i = 1, ..., K. \tag{4.16}$$

The CA trend test statistic is calculated as

$$X_{CA}^2 = \left[\frac{\sum_{i=1}^{K} (d_i - \bar{d}) s_i}{\sqrt{\bar{\pi}(1 - \bar{\pi}) \sum_{i=1}^{K} n_i (d_i - \bar{d})^2}} \right]^2, \tag{4.17}$$

where $\bar{d} = \sum_i n_i d_i / \sum_i n_i$ is the average dose level and $\bar{\pi} = \sum_i s_i / \sum_i n_i$ is the average ADA response rate. Under the null hypothesis, X_{CA}^2 follows a chi-square distribution with $DF = 1$. The null hypothesis of equal ADA response rates is rejected when $X_{CA}^2 \geq \chi_1^2(1 - \alpha)$.

Another popular model for the response probabilities $\pi_i, i = 1, ..., K$ is the logistic model.

$$\log \left(\frac{\pi_i}{1 - \pi_i} \right) = \alpha + \beta d_i. \tag{4.18}$$

TABLE 4.3
Number and percentage of ADA+ patients by treatment group

Dose Group	# of patients	# ADA +	% of ADA+	95% CI	
Placebo	150	8	5.3	2.7	10.4
10 mg	150	25	16.7	11.5	23.6
20 mg	150	40	26.7	20.1	34.4
40 mg	150	60	40.0	32.4	48.1

The null hypothesis of equal response probability can be formulated as H_0 : $\beta = 0$ and the alternative hypothesis of increasing trend is equivalent to $H_1 : \beta > 0$. The logistic model and the Wald-test of zero slope can be fitted using SAS PROC LOGISTIC or R function *glm*. The advantage of a logistic model is that multiple explanatory variables other than dose level can be included to avoid the confounding effects of other variables in equation (4.18).

As discussed in Chapter 1, the propensity of inducing immunogenicity could depend on both product-related risk factors and patient-specific characteristics. For example, prior exposure to the similar product may increase the immunogenicity and concomitant medication may alter the patients' ADA response. Certain genetic makeups may predispose patients to development of undesirable ADA responses to specific products (Hoffmann et al. (2008)).

4.3.5   Example

In the hypothetical clinical trial consisting of 600 RA patients, 150 patients were randomly assigned into each of the four dose groups. The ADA responses of the patients are summarized in Table 4.3. The ADA+ cases included both prevalent and incident cases. The percentages of ADA+ increased with dose levels with a maximum of 40.0% in the 40mg group. The estimates of OR and RR for comparing the ADA response rates between the treated groups and the placebo group are shown in Table 4.4. For example, the odds of having ADA+ in the 10mg dose group is 3.55 fold over the odds in the placebo group with a 95% CI is (1.5454, 8.1546). The value of OR increases with dose, indicating a dose-response trend. In general, the estimates of OR are greater than those of RR. When the response rates are small, the OR is a close approximation of the RR. When the response rates are high, the OR tends to over estimate the RR.

To further examine the statistical significance of the differences in the ADA response rates, both Pearson's chi-square test and Fisher's exact test were performed. The test *p*-values are shown in Table 4.5. All tests were highly significant with *p*-values less than 0.01. These results indicate that the ADA response rates for all three dose groups are significantly different from

TABLE 4.4
Estimates of OR and RR of ADA responses between the treatment groups and the placebo group

Dose Group	Risk Measure	Estimate	95% CI	
10 mg	Odds Ratio	3.5500	1.5454	8.1546
10 mg	Risk Ratio	3.1250	1.4566	6.7042
20 mg	Odds Ratio	6.4545	2.9035	14.3486
20 mg	Risk Ratio	5.0000	2.4227	10.3192
40 mg	Odds Ratio	11.8333	5.4053	25.9058
40 mg	Risk Ratio	7.5000	3.7165	15.1354

TABLE 4.5
Statistical tests that compare the ADA response rates between the treatment groups and the placebo group

Dose Group	Statistic	*p*-value
10 mg	Chi-square	0.0017
10 mg	Fisher's exact test	0.0027
20 mg	Chi-square	<.0001
20 mg	Fisher's exact test	<.0001
40 mg	Chi-Square	<.0001
40 mg	Fisher's exact test	<.0001

the ADA response rate of the placebo group. In addition, the CA trend test statistic is $X^2_{CA} = 56.6$ with p-value< 0.0001, showing an upward trend in the percentages of ADA+ subjects with respect to dose level.

4.4 Effects of ADA on Drug Efficacy

Most clinical trials are conducted to evaluate the efficacy of novel drugs. In a clinical trial, a clinical endpoint should directly and indirectly measure how a patient feels, functions or survives. A clinical endpoint should be a valid reflection of the drug's true effectiveness in treating the disease, or alleviating some or all of the symptoms caused by the disease. Typical endpoints with subjective measures include disease symptom scores, self evaluation, and quality-of-life measures. In the majority of clinical trials, efficacy is assessed using on objective measures, e.g., overall survival (OS), progression-free survival (PFS), laboratory test or validated biomarkers.

The choice of efficacy endpoints for a new drug is highly specific to the drug, disease, and the objective of the clinical trial. A valid endpoint should satisfy the following qualitative criteria (Riegelman and Hirsch (1989)):

• should be an measure of a response that is directly relevant to the clinical benefit of the drug.

• should be an accurate and unbiased measure of disease status by combining information from supplementary test, assessment and reports.

• should be based on enough data from a sufficient number of patients.

• should be reliable and not sensitive to data collection method.

In "Guideline on clinical investigation of medicinal products other than NSAIDs for treatment of RA" (EMA (2006)), the European Medicines Agency (EMA) recommends that clinical trials for treatment of RA include the following goals:

• relief of symptoms, e.g., pain

• achievement of remission/low disease activity state

• decrease of inflammatory synovitis

• improvement or sustainment of physical function

• prevention or slowing of structural joint damage.

The goals should be assessed by validated and objective measures and/or scores. As such, we chose remission of RA as the primary endpoints and the composite DAS28 score as the secondary endpoint. Here, we focus on the effect of ADA responses on efficacy. As illustrated in Figure 4.1, treatment group (X) is the primary factor that is related to efficacy (Y). The formation of ADA (Z) may alter or mediate the effect of treatment on clinical endpoints. If we are interested in the effect of ADA response Z on efficacy measure Y, the treatment should be treated as a confounding factor. As described in early chapters, most biologics induce ADA responses that in some cases may cause AEs, and/or reduced drug efficacy. Thus, monitoring of ADA responses and risk assessment are required in clinical trials for biologics.

4.4.1   Categorical Endpoints as Efficacy Measure

In a clinical trial, primary and secondary endpoints can be nominal or ordinal categorical variables. The simplest case of a nominal endpoint is the binary response, i.e., responders or non-responders of RA treatment according to the pre-defined criteria. The endpoint may be ordinal variable, for example, the improvement of RA symptoms categorized as no improvement, moderate improvement, remarkable improvement, or the score of various standard joint counts (Felson et al. (1998)).

4.4.1.1   Multiple 2×2 Tables

If both treatment and ADA response are associated with efficacy, the effect of immunogenicity on efficacy should be estimated after controlling for the possible confounding effect of other factors including treatment dose. For binary efficacy endpoint, the data are stratified into multiple 2×2 tables. Suppose that the stratification variable is the treatment doses $x_k, k = 1, ..., K$ and x_k is the dose level for the kth stratum. For the kth stratum, the 2×2 table for the binary ADA response and clinical endpoint is summarized in Table 4.6.

TABLE 4.6
The 2×2 table of ADA status and clinical response in the kth dose group

Clinical endpoint	ADA $+$	ADA $-$	
$+$	s_{k1}	s_{k2}	m_{k1}
$-$	$n_{k1} - s_{k1}$	$n_{k2} - s_{k2}$	m_{k2}
All	n_{k1}	n_{k2}	n_k

One of the most popular methods for stratified $K \times 2 \times 2$ contingency table is the Cochran–Mantel–Haenszel (CMH) test (Cochran (1954b); Mantel and Haenszel (1959)). The CMH test is a nonparametric test, and is also related to the logistic model.

For the kth stratum, let $\pi_{ik} = P(Y = 1 | Z = i, X = k), i = 0, 1, k = 1, ..., K$ be the response probability of a positive clinical response Y for an

ADA response Z for the kth dose group. We consider a logit model

$$\text{logit}(\pi_{ik}) = \alpha + \beta Z + \gamma_k^X, \tag{4.19}$$

where $Z = 0$ for ADA$-$ and $Z = 1$ means ADA$+$. The odds ratio of ADA response on the binary efficacy endpoint is calculated as $\exp(\beta)$. This model assumes that the odds ratios of Z on Y are the same across different dose levels. Cochran (1954b) and Mantel and Haenszel (1959) considered the CMH test for multiple conditionally independent 2×2 tables in a retrospective study design. The CMH test statistic can be calculated as

$$T_{CMH} = \frac{\left[\sum_{k=1}^{K}(s_{k1} - \mu_{k1})\right]^2}{\sum_{k=1}^{K} \text{Var}(s_{k1})}, \tag{4.20}$$

where μ_{k1} and $\text{Var}(s_{k1})$ are the mean and variance of s_{k1}:

$$
\begin{aligned}
\mu_{k1} &= E(s_{k1}) = m_{k1}n_{k1}/n_k \\
\text{Var}(s_{k1}) &= m_{k1}m_{k2}n_{k1}n_{k2}/n_k^2(n_k - 1).
\end{aligned}
$$

Under the null hypothesis of no ADA effect on efficacy, i.e., $H_0 : \beta = 0$, the test statistic T_{CMH} follows a Chi-square distribution with $DF = 1$ for large sample size. The CMH test works well when the effects of ADA are similar for each treatment group or stratum.

Westfall et al. (2002) proposed a permutation test for the stratified Mantel–Haenszel test, which permuted the two-sample binary data within each stratum in the context of multiple testing. Jung (2014) provided a less computation-intensive Fisher's exact test for multiple 2×2 tables. The homogeneity of the odds ratios from different strata can be tested using the methods proposed by Cochran (1954a), Zelen (1971), and Breslow and Day (1987). For other tests used for multiple 2×2 tables, see Lachin (2014).

4.4.1.2 Multiple $R \times C$ Tables

The clinical endpoint could be a categorical variable with more than two levels. For example, the efficacy endpoint in the RA trial could be improvement of RA symptoms, which is classified as "no improvement," "slight improvement," "marked improvement." Using treatment dose as the control variable, the data for the effect of ADA on efficacy can be summarized as multiple $R \times C$ tables (Agresti (2014)). Let Z be the binary indicator for the ADA response.

For ordinal efficacy endpoint $Y \in \{1, ..., J\}$, the model can be specified as

$$\text{logit}[P(Y \le j|Z, X = k)] = \alpha_j + \beta Z + \gamma_k^X. \tag{4.21}$$

The null hypothesis of no ADA effect on efficacy is equivalent to $H_0 : \beta = 0$. A large-sample Chi-square test can be derived from the likelihood ratio test, score test or Wald test statistics under the null hypothesis (Agresti (2014)).

TABLE 4.7
RA recurrence status by ADA status and dose level

			RA recurrence	
Dose Group	ADA Response	All	No Recurrence	Recurrence
Placebo	No	142	105	37
	Yes	8	6	2
10 mg	No	125	94	31
	Yes	25	16	9
20 mg	No	110	94	16
	Yes	40	34	6
40 mg	No	90	75	15
	Yes	60	48	12

For nominal efficacy endpoints with J unordered categories, the model with level J as the reference level can be specified as

$$\log \left[\frac{P(Y = j | Z, X = k)}{P(Y = J | Z, X = k)} \right] = \alpha_{jk} + \beta_j Z, j = 1, ..., J - 1. \qquad (4.22)$$

The null hypothesis of no ADA effect on efficacy is formulated as $H_0 : \beta_1 = \cdots = \beta_{J-1} = 0$ versus $H_1 :$ at least one $\beta_j \neq 0$. A large-sample Chi-square test has $df = J - 1$.

4.4.1.3 Example

In the RA trial, the patients were followed up for the recurrence of symptoms. The efficacy endpoint was defined as a binary indicator of RA recurrence. To examine the effect of ADA on RA recurrence, the data are stratified by dose level and summarized into $4 \times 2 \times 2$ table in Table 4.7.

The Breslow–Day test of the homogeneity for the odds ratios across multiple strata is a Chi-square test with $DF = 3$. The homogeneity test statistic is 0.6821 with p-value 0.8774 and the CMH test statistic is 0.8803 with p-value 0.3481. Therefore, the odds ratios of ADA on recurrence are homogeneous across different dose groups and the ADA response rates increase significantly with the dose level. However, the occurrence of ADA reaction seems not related to the RA recurrence.

4.4.2 Effect of ADA on Survival Outcomes

In many clinical trials, patients are followed up for a certain period of time after administration of the last dose to monitor the disease progression and to evaluate efficacy and safety. The focus of these studies is on the time when the event of interest occurs, e.g., death, relapse, AE or development of a secondary disease. For the clinical trials of RA, a typical endpoint is the time from the beginning of the study to recurrence of RA symptoms. The follow-up time for the study may vary from a few days to many years. Survival analysis is generally defined as a suite of methods for analyzing data of time-to-event of interest. Therefore, the survival analysis is also called time-to-event analysis. As time-to-event is a very important endpoint in many clinical trials, survival analysis is a very popular tool in clinical research and provides invaluable information about the drug effect.

A different set of statistical techniques are used to analyze the time-to-event data because survival time is different from the typical outcomes. First, survival times can only take positive values and the usual regression models based on normal distributions may not be suitable for positive-only outcomes. More importantly, censoring, a phenomenon that the event times of patients without events of interest cannot be exactly observed, is common in survival analysis. The main references for survival analysis include Cox and Oakes (1984), Lawless (1982), Ibrahim et al. (2001), Kalbfleisch and Prentice (2002), Klein and Moeschberger (2003), and Fleming and Harrington (2011).

Let T denote time from a specific origin to an event of interest. While T may not be the survival time until death, we still use the term "survival time" to denote the time to event. The basic function that describes the distribution of survival time T is the survival function

$$S(t) = \Pr(T > t), \tag{4.23}$$

which is the probability of a subject surviving beyond time t. If T is a continuous random variable, then the survival function $S(t) = 1 - F(t)$, where $F(t) = \Pr(T \leq t)$ is the cumulative distribution function. Let $f(x)$ denote the probability density function, i.e., $f(t) = \frac{\mathrm{d}F(t)}{\mathrm{d}t}$. One important measure in survival analysis is the instant hazard function $\lambda(t)$, which is defined as the event rate at time t conditional on survival until time t or later. For continuous survival times, the hazard function is calculated as

$$\lambda(t) = \lim_{\Delta t \to 0} \frac{\Pr(t \leq T < t + \Delta t | T \geq t)}{\Delta t} = \frac{f(t)}{S(t)} = -\frac{\mathrm{d}\log S(t)}{\mathrm{d}x}. \tag{4.24}$$

In demography and actuarial science, a synonym of the hazard function is force of mortality. The hazard function can alternatively be represented in terms of the cumulative hazard function, which is defined as

$$\Lambda(t) = \int_0^t \lambda(s)\mathrm{d}s = -\log S(t). \tag{4.25}$$

Based on the definition of $\Lambda(t)$, it increases without bound as $t \to \infty$ if $\lim_{t \to \infty} S(t) = 0$. This implies that $\lambda(t)$ must not decrease too quickly, since, by definition, the cumulative hazard function is a divergent function.

Survival times are censored when the exact event times are not observed, but known to be within a certain range. The two most common types of censoring are the right censoring and the interval censoring. Often times, right censoring occurs when the study ends and some subjects have not experienced failure yet or some individuals dropped out or were lost to follow-up during the study. The available information is that these individuals are still free of the event at the last observation time C, i.e., $T > C$. The other type of censoring occurs when the failure time is known to occur only within a certain interval. For example, in a clinical trial or a longitudinal study where the patients are followed up periodically, a patient who does not have the failure right before time L but failed before time R is interval censored $[L, R)$. Therefore, the event time T is interval-censored, i.e., $T \in (L, R]$. A special case of interval censoring is left-censoring. For instance, in a pediatric study of acute otitis media (middle-ear infection), the enrolled children will be monitored to determine the children's age when they have the first event of acute otitis media. Often, some children have already had the mid-ear infection before the age at enrollment L (Andreev and Arjas (1998)). Therefore, the onset age T is left censored at age L.

Another feature of survival data, which is often confused with censoring is called *truncation* (Klein and Moeschberger (2003)). Truncation occurs when some subjects who may experience the event of interest are not included in the study, e.g., ineligible for the study or dying prior to the study initiation. Under these circumstances, the subjects are not considered the population at risk. For example, in a longitudinal cohort study where all subjects in a community are followed up to ascertain the status of cancer onset, the subjects who died before the beginning of the study are not included in the study. Therefore, we don't know whether those excluded subjects had cancer or not. This phenomenon is also called *delayed entry* (Keiding (2005)). As opposed to left censoring, where we know that the event of interests occur prior to certain age at enrollment. For instance, in the otitis media study, the left-truncated individuals were never included in the analysis.

Here, we consider the estimation and test for continuous survival times with right censoring and left truncation. Let $t_1 < t_2 < \cdots < t_K$ denote K distinct event times for the study sample. At time t_i there are d_i failures and the number of subjects at risk at time t_i is Y_i. The number of people at risk at t_i are the number of people who are still alive right before time t_i. The survival function $S(t)$ can be estimated by the Kaplan–Meier or the product-limit estimator (Kaplan and Meier (1958)):

$$\hat{S}_{KM}(t) = \begin{cases} 1 & \text{if } t < t_1 \\ \prod_{t_i < t}(1 - \frac{d_i}{Y_i}) & \text{if } t \geq t_1 \end{cases}. \tag{4.26}$$

If there are failures at the last observation time, we usually set $\hat{S}(t) = 0$ for $t > t_K$. If the last observed time is censored, the value of $\hat{S}(t)$ is not well defined for $t > t_K$. Gill (1980) suggested setting $\hat{S}(t) = \hat{S}(t_K)$ for $t > t_K$, which assumes that all the survivors at time t_K would not die when $t < \infty$. This estimator is positively biased, but it converges to the true survival function for large samples (Klein and Moeschberger (2003)). Greenwood's formula is often used to estimate the variance of the Kaplan–Meier estimator

$$\hat{V}[\hat{S}(t)] = \hat{S}(t)^2 \sum_{t_i \leq t} \frac{d_i}{Y_i(Y_i - d_i)}. \tag{4.27}$$

4.4.2.1 Rank-Based Statistical Tests

Log-rank test and related rank-based tests are often used to compare the survival distributions of two or multiple samples. The rank-based statistical tests are a class of nonparametric tests that are appropriate for right-skewed and censored data. The goal of the rank-based method in clinical trials is to test the difference of survival distributions in the control and treatment groups. For a two-sample test, the hypothesis is $H_0 : S_1(t) = S_2(t)$ for all $t > 0$ versus $H_1 : S_1(t) \neq S_2(t)$ for some t. For right-censored data, the rank-based methods use the rankings within the combined sample to test whether the different samples come from the same population. The most commonly used test to compare survival functions is the log-rank test.

The two-sample survival data typically consists of independent right-censored survival times from two groups. In the analysis of immunogenicity, the two groups are the ADA+ and the ADA− groups. Let $t_1 < t_2 < \cdots < t_K$ be K distinct observed failure times. At time t_i, we observed d_{ij} number of events among the Y_{ij} number of subjects at risk in group $j, j = 1, 2$. The total number of people at risk right before time t_i is $Y_i = Y_{i1} + Y_{i2}$ and the total number of events at time t_i is $d_i = d_{i1} + d_{i2}$. For right-censored survival data, the log-rank test is equivalent to the score test for the proportional hazards regression model. We consider the problem of comparing the hazard functions of two groups:

$$H_0 : \lambda_1(t) = \lambda_2(t) \text{ for all } t \leq \tau, \text{ vs } H_1 : \lambda_1(t) \neq \lambda_2(t) \text{ for some } t \leq \tau. \tag{4.28}$$

Under the null hypothesis of equal hazard functions or survival functions, the mean and variance of d_{i1} are

$$E(d_{i1}) = d_i \frac{Y_{i1}}{Y_i},$$

$$\text{Var}(d_{i1}) = \frac{Y_{i1}Y_{i2}d_i(Y_i - d_i)}{Y_i^2(Y_i - 1)}.$$

The log-rank test statistical is calculated as

$$T_{LR} = \frac{\sum_{i=1}^{K}[d_{i1} - E(d_{i1})]}{\sqrt{\sum_{i=1}^{K} \text{Var}(d_{i1})}} = \frac{\sum_{i=1}^{K}\left[d_{i1} - d_i \frac{Y_{i1}}{Y_i}\right]}{\sqrt{\sum_{i=1}^{K} \frac{Y_{i1}Y_{i2}d_i(Y_i - d_i)}{Y_i^2(Y_i - 1)}}}. \tag{4.29}$$

Under the null hypothesis, T_{LR} follows an asymptotic standard normal distribution for large samples. The log-rank test is the optimal test for detecting alternative hypothesis under the assumption that the hazard rates for the two groups are proportional to each other. In general, the rank-type test statistic is calculated as

$$T_W = \frac{\sum_{i=1}^{K} W_i \left[d_{i1} - d_i \frac{Y_{i1}}{Y_i} \right]}{\sqrt{\sum_{i=1}^{K} W_i^2 \frac{Y_{i1} Y_{i2} d_i (Y_i - d_i)}{Y_i^2 (Y_i - 1)}}}. \tag{4.30}$$

where $W_i = W(t_i)$ is the weight function. A variety of weight functions have been proposed to accommodate different assumptions about hazard functions (Klein and Moeschberger (2003)). The rank-based tests have been implemented in most statistical packages, e.g., PROC LIFETEST in SAS.

In the analysis of immunogenicity, the focus is the effect of ADA responses on survival outcomes after controlling for the effects of other confounding factors. The confounding factors, e.g., treatment or dose level, can be used for stratification. Suppose that there are M treatment groups. The statistical testing of ADA effect on survival can be formulated as

$$H_0 : \lambda_{1m}(t) = \lambda_{2m}(t), \text{ for all } m = 1, ..., M, t < \tau \tag{4.31}$$

versus

$$H_1 : \lambda_{1m}(t) \neq \lambda_{2m}(t) \text{ for some } t \text{ and } m. \tag{4.32}$$

For the mth stratum, let $t_1^{(m)} < t_2^{(m)} < \cdots < t_K^{(m)}$ be K distinct observed failure times and let $d_{ij}^{(m)}$ be the number of events among the $Y_{ij}^{(m)}$ number of subjects at risk in group $j, j = 1, 2$. The total number of people at risk right before time $t_i^{(m)}$ is $Y_i^{(m)} = Y_{i1}^{(m)} + Y_{i2}^{(m)}$ and the total number of events at time $t_i^{(m)}$ is $d_i^{(m)} = d_{i1}^{(m)} + d_{i2}^{(m)}$. The stratified long-rank test (T_{SLR}) is analogous to the CMH test after adjustment for stratification factor:

$$T_{SLR} = \frac{\sum_{m=1}^{M} \sum_{i=1}^{K} [d_{i1}^{(m)} - E(d_{i1}^{(m)})]}{\sqrt{\sum_{i=1}^{K} \text{Var}(d_{i1}^{(m)})}}. \tag{4.33}$$

4.4.2.2 Survival Regression Models

Nonparametric methods are useful to compare the survival distributions among two or more groups. Stratification can be used to control the effects of confounding factors. In general, the subjects under study may have some additional characteristics other than the treatment that may be related to efficacy. For example, the demographic variables like age, gender, education have been shown to be related to longevity. Comorbidity, smoking history, and the genetic makeup of cancer patients are important factors for the cancer prognosis. These variables may be confounding factors for the development of ADA. Excluding them from the analysis of immunogenicity effect may lead to biased and less precise estimates of ADA effect on efficacy. Regression models are often used to assess the effect of ADA on survival outcomes in the presence of confounding factors. We will focus on the widely used multiplicative hazards model introduced by Cox (1972). This type of model is often called the Cox proportional hazards model.

The Cox proportional hazards model assumes that the hazard function is a multiplicative function of covariates:

$$\lambda(t|X) = \lambda_0(t)\exp(\boldsymbol{\beta}'\boldsymbol{X}), \qquad t \geq 0 \tag{4.34}$$

where $\lambda_0(t)$ is the baseline hazard function, $\boldsymbol{X}$ is the vector of covariates and $\boldsymbol{\beta}$ is the vector of regression coefficients. Typically, the survival data consists of $(t_i, \delta_i, \boldsymbol{X}_i), i = 1, ..., n$, where t_i is the observed event or censoring time, δ_i is the indicator of failure ($\delta_i = 1$ means event and $\delta_i = 0$ means censoring) and $\boldsymbol{X}_i = (X_{i1}, X_{i2}, ..., X_{ip})'$ is a p-dimensional vector of covariates for the ith subject. We assume that the event times and the censoring times are independent.

The likelihood function for the survival data $\{(t_i, \delta_i, \boldsymbol{X}_i), i = 1, ..., n\}$ can be written as

$$L(\boldsymbol{\beta}, \lambda_0) = \lambda_0(t_i)^{\delta_i}\exp(\delta_i\boldsymbol{\beta}'\boldsymbol{X}_i)\exp\left(-\int_0^{t_i}\lambda_0(s)\exp(\boldsymbol{\beta}'\boldsymbol{X}_i)ds\right). \tag{4.35}$$

However, the maximization of the full likelihood $L(\boldsymbol{\beta}, \lambda_0)$ cannot be handled because of the infinite dimensional nuisance parameter $\lambda_0(t)$. To solve this problem, Cox (1972) proposed the partial likelihood method for the estimation of the β's. Alternatively, Breslow (1974) suggested an estimator for the cumulative hazard $\Lambda_0(t) = \int_0^t \lambda_0(s)ds$.

Under the assumption that there are no ties of the event times, let $\tau_1 < \tau_2 < \cdots < \tau_D$ denote the distinct event times and let $\boldsymbol{X}_{(j)}$ denote the covariates for the subject whose failure time is τ_j. The risk set at time τ_j, denoted as $R(\tau_j)$, is defined as the set of all subjects who are still free of events at time just prior to τ_j. The partial likelihood function (Cox (1972)) is specified as

$$PL(\boldsymbol{\beta}) = \prod_{j=1}^{D}\frac{\exp(\boldsymbol{\beta}'\boldsymbol{X}_{(j)})}{\sum_{l\in R(\tau_j)}\exp(\boldsymbol{\beta}'\boldsymbol{X}_l)}. \tag{4.36}$$

The MLE of $\boldsymbol{\beta}$ can be obtained by maximizing the partial likelihood $PL(\boldsymbol{\beta})$.

Another common approach to survival analysis is the accelerated failure time (AFT) model. The AFT model assumes that the logarithm of the survival times is associated with the covariates via a linear regression model,

$$\log(T) = \alpha + \boldsymbol{\beta}'\boldsymbol{X} + \sigma W, \tag{4.37}$$

where α is the intercept, $\boldsymbol{X}$ is the vector of covariates, $\boldsymbol{\beta}$ is the vector of corresponding regression coefficients, σ is the scale parameter and W is the error term. The common choice for the error distributions for W include the standard normal distribution, extreme value distribution and the log-logistic distributions. The resulting distributions of the survival time are the lognormal, Weibull and logistic distributions, respectively. Let $S_0(t)$ be the survival function of T when $\boldsymbol{X} = 0$, i.e., $S_0(t)$ is the survival function of $\exp(\mu + \sigma W)$. Then

$$\Pr(T > t|\boldsymbol{X}) = \Pr(\mu + \sigma W > \log t - \boldsymbol{\beta}'\boldsymbol{X}|\boldsymbol{X}) = S_0(\exp(-\boldsymbol{\beta}'\boldsymbol{X})t). \quad (4.38)$$

Depending on the sign of $\boldsymbol{\beta}'\boldsymbol{X}$, the time t in the survival function is either accelerated or decelerated by a constant factor. The corresponding hazard function of an AFT model is

$$\lambda(t|\boldsymbol{X}) = \lambda_0(t \exp(-\boldsymbol{\beta}'\boldsymbol{X}))\exp(-\boldsymbol{\beta}'\boldsymbol{X}). \quad (4.39)$$

The estimation of the AFT models and the Cox models has been implemented in SAS PROC LIFEREG and PROC PHREG and R function *survreg*.

4.4.2.3 Recurrent Event Data

Multivariate survival data arise when each study subject has multiple or recurrent events that are inter-dependent or the event times come from multiple individuals in the same cluster or group. For chronic diseases, recurrent events are common. Typical examples include tumor recurrence for cancer patients; multiple relapses from remission for leukemia patients; repeated episodes of otitis media. A popular model that capture the association between multiple recurrent events for the same subjects is the frailty (random-effects) model. A frailty is actually a random effect that is shared by the recurrent events of the same subject.

We assume a proportional hazards model for each individual recurrent event. For the ith subject, the n_i recurrent events share the common random-effect b_i. The hazard rate of the jth recurrent event for the ith subject can be written as

$$\lambda_{ij}(t) = \lambda_0(t)\exp\left(\boldsymbol{\beta}'\boldsymbol{X}_{ij} + \delta b_i\right), \quad (4.40)$$

where $\lambda_0(t)$ is the baseline hazard function, $\boldsymbol{\beta}$ is the vector of regression coefficients, $\boldsymbol{X}_{ij}$ is the covariates for the ith subject at jth recurrent event time, b_i is the common random-effect associated with the ith subject. Usually, we assume that $E(b_i) = 0$ and $\text{Var}(b_i) = 1$. Let $u_i = \exp(b_i)$. The rescaled random-effects u_i's are often called the frailty. Common distributions for the frailty include the gamma distribution (Clayton (1978)), the lognormal distribution (McGilchrist and Aisbett (1991)), and the positive stable distribution (Hougaard (1986)). As an illustration, we present the Clayton's frailty model, where the frailty terms u_i's follow a gamma distribution:

$$g(u) = \frac{u^{\frac{1}{\gamma}-1}\exp\left(-\frac{u}{\gamma}\right)}{\Gamma(\frac{1}{\gamma})\gamma^{\frac{1}{\gamma}}}. \quad (4.41)$$

The gamma frailty model was initially used by Clayton in a copula model

(Clayton (1978)). The mean and the variance of the gamma frailty are 1 and γ, respectively. A larger value of γ indicates a greater degree of heterogeneity.

Let the n_i recurrent event times for the ith subject be denoted as $t_{i1}, ..., t_{in_i}$. The observed survival data consist of $(t_{ij}, \delta_{ij}, \boldsymbol{X}_{ij}), j = 1, ..., n_i, i = 1, ..., n$. The joint survival function for the n_i recurrent event times is given by

$$S(t_{i1}, ..., t_{in_1}) = \mathrm{P}(T_{i1} > t_{i1}, \cdots, T_{in_i} > t_{in_i}) = \left[1 + \gamma \sum_{j=1}^{n_i} \Lambda_0(t_{ij}) \exp(\boldsymbol{\beta}' \boldsymbol{X}_{ij}) \right]^{-\frac{1}{\gamma}}.$$

where $\Lambda_0(t) = \int_0^t \lambda(s)\mathrm{d}s$ is the baseline cumulative hazard function.

The log-likelihood function for the observed survival data is

$$\begin{aligned}
L(\boldsymbol{\beta}, \gamma) &= \sum_{i=1}^{n} D_i \log \gamma + \log \left(\frac{\Gamma(D_i + 1/\gamma)}{\Gamma(1/\gamma)} \right) \\
&+ \left(D_i + \frac{1}{\gamma} \right) \log \left[1 + \gamma \sum_{j=1}^{n_i} H_0(t_{ij}) \exp(\boldsymbol{\beta}' \boldsymbol{X}_{ij}) \right] \\
&+ \sum_{j=1}^{n_i} \delta_{ij} [\boldsymbol{\beta}' \boldsymbol{X}_{ij} + \log \lambda_0(t_i j)],
\end{aligned} \tag{4.42}$$

where $D_i = \sum_{j=1}^{n_i} \delta_{ij}$ is the number of total recurrent events for the ith subject.

If a parametric model is used for $\lambda_0(t)$, the MLEs can be obtained by directly maximizing the loglikelihoood (4.42). When the baseline hazard $\lambda_0(t)$ is not specified, this leads to a semi-parametric proportional hazards gamma-frailty model. The parameter estimates can be obtained using an expectation-maximization (EM) algorithm (Dempster et al. (1977)) by treating the frailty u_i's as missing data (Andersen et al. (1997); Klein and Moeschberger (2003)). The parameter estimates can also be obtained using the penalized likelihood method (Rondeau et al. (2003)). The penalized likelihood (PL) function is defined as:

$$PL(\boldsymbol{\beta}, \gamma) = L(\boldsymbol{\beta}, \gamma) + \kappa \int_0^\infty \lambda_0''^2(t)\mathrm{d}t, \tag{4.43}$$

where $L(\boldsymbol{\beta}, \gamma)$ is the log-likelihood function (4.42), $\lambda_0''(t)$ is the second derivative of the baseline hazard function $\lambda_0(t)$, and κ is a positive parameter that controls the smoothness of the baseline hazard function $\lambda_0(t)$. The maximum penalized likelihood estimators can obtained using an iterative algorithm (Rondeau et al. (2012)). The penalized likelihood method has been implemented in R package `frailtypack` and SAS macro (Shu (1997)). The parameter estimates from the penalized likelihood method are the MLE for the gamma frailty model and approximate MLE for the lognormal model. Compared to the EM algorithm, the penalized likelihood method has simple computation and faster convergence. The disadvantage of the penalized likelihood method is that it is difficult to obtain a valid estimate of the standard error of the frailty parameter γ. A modified EM algorithm for the shared Gamma frailty models was proposed to handle data sets with large number of clusters and distinct event times (Yu (2006)).

4.4.2.4 Competing-Risks Survival Data

The competing-risks survival data arise when the study subjects are at risk of having multiple types of events, e.g., cancer recurrence and death are two types of dependent, but often distinct outcomes in a cancer clinical trial. Oftentimes, occurrence of an event other than the one of interest may alter the probability of experiencing the event of interest. For example, a cancer patient who dies from heart attack will no longer have the risk of cancer recurrence. Therefore, the analysis methods for competing-risk survival data are usually different from those for clustered or recurrent event data.

Let the cause of death $D = k$ denote the kth event type, $k = 1, ..., K$, and T be the actual time of any event and X be the associated covariate vector. When the subject is still event-free at time t, then the subject is censored at time t. The censored observation is denoted as $D = 0$. The cause-specific hazard function for cause k at time t is expressed as

$$\lambda_k(t) = \lim_{\Delta t \to 0} \frac{\Pr(t \leq T < t + \Delta t, D = k | T \geq t)}{\Delta t}. \qquad (4.44)$$

The simplest case is that there is only one cause of death. In an oncology trial, overall survival (OS) is often used as an efficacy endpoint and all other non-death events are not considered as events.

The cumulative incidence function for the kth event, denoted by $F_k(t)$, is the probability of failure due to cause k prior to time t. It is calculated as

$$F_k(t) = \Pr(T \leq t, D = k), k = 1, ..., K. \qquad (4.45)$$

The cumulative incidence function $F_k(t)$ is also referred to as the subdistribution function because it is not a true probability distribution. Following the definition (4.45), we obtain

$$F_k(t) = \int_0^t S(u)\lambda_k(u)\mathrm{d}u. \qquad (4.46)$$

Let $\Lambda_k(t) = \int_0^t \lambda_k(u)\mathrm{d}u$ denote the cause-specific cumulative hazard function and let $S(t) = \Pr(T > t) = \exp(-\sum_{k=1}^{K} \Lambda_k(t))$ be the overall survival function.

Let $t_1 < t_2 < \cdots < t_j < \cdots < t_n$ be the distinct event times from any cause, the cumulative hazard function for cause k can be estimated by the Nelson–Aalen estimator (Borgan (2005))

$$\hat{\Lambda}_k(t) = \sum_{t_j \leq t} \frac{d_{kj}}{n_j} \qquad (4.47)$$

where d_{kj} is the number of failures from cause k and n_j is the number of subjects at risk at time t_j. The overall survival function $S(t)$ can be estimated from the Kaplan–Meier estimator. After plugging these two estimators into the equation for $F_k(t)$, the cumulative incidence function for cause k can be estimated as (Marubini and Valsecchi (2004))

$$\hat{F}_k(t) = \sum_{t_j \leq t} \hat{S}(t_{j-1}) \frac{d_{kj}}{n_j}. \tag{4.48}$$

Note that $\hat{F}_k(t)$ is a step function that changes only at failure times t_j where $d_{kj} > 0$. For survival data with only one cause of failure, there is a one-to-one relationship between the hazard function and the survival function. This is not the case in the presence of competing risks. Based on the definition of $F_k(t)$, the subdistribution function is related to all cause-specific hazard functions through $S(t)$. Therefore, $F_k(t)$ is not defined solely by $\lambda_k(t)$.

Using the delta method, the variance of the cumulative incidence function estimate $\hat{F}_k(t)$ can be derived as

$$\text{Var}(\hat{F}_k(t)) = \sum_{t_j \leq t} \left\{ [\hat{F}_k(t) - \hat{F}_k(t_j)]^2 \right\} \frac{d_j}{n_j(n_j - d_j)}$$
$$+ [\hat{S}(t_{j-1})]^2 \frac{n_j - d_{kj}}{n_j^3} - 2[\hat{F}_k(t) - \hat{F}_k(t_j)]\hat{S}(t_{j-1}) \frac{d_{kj}}{n_j},$$

where $d_j = \sum_{k=1}^{k} d_{kj}$. The associated CIs can be computed directly from $\hat{F}_k(t)$ and its variance $\text{Var}(\hat{F}_k(t))$.

4.4.2.5 Example

In Section 4.4.1, the CMH test showed that the existence of ADA response did not change the recurrence rate of the RA symptoms. Survival analysis allows us to examine whether occurrence of ADA has an impact on the time to the recurrence of RA symptoms. First, the Kaplan–Meier curves for the ADA+ and ADA− subjects for all dose groups combined were plotted (Figure 4.2). For both the ADA− and ADA+ groups, about 76% subjects remain under remission after one year. The recurrence for the ADA+ group is slightly higher than the ADA− group in early follow-up time.

To understand the effect of ADA on time to RA recurrence after controlling for the dose level, the Kaplan–Meier curves of percent of subjects in remission over time for each of the four dose groups were plotted (Figure 4.3). As expected, a low percentage of subjects in the placebo group were ADA+ (5% of the 150 subjects). Because the placebo has no active pharmaceutical ingredient (API), the positive ADA responses were likely either false-positives or ADA responses to one or more of the product excipients. We also see some early differences of the Kaplan–Meier curves for the treated groups. After controlling for the dose level, the stratified log-rank test statistic is $T^2_{SLR} = 1.4$

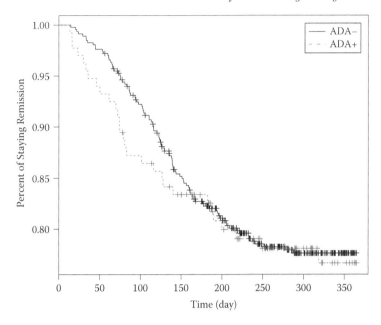

FIGURE 4.2
Kaplan–Meier estimates of % of subjects staying in remission by ADA status.

with p-value=0.237 (Table 4.8). While prior to day 150, there were differences in the remission rate based on ADA status, overall the differences were not statistically significant.

To quantify the effect of ADA and dose level on the hazard of RA recurrence, we fit a Cox regression model with both ADA status and dose level as covariates:

$$\lambda(t|\boldsymbol{x}) = \lambda_0(t) \exp(\beta_1 x_1 + \beta_2 x_2), \qquad (4.49)$$

ADA status (x_1) is a binary variable and dose level (x_2) is an ordinal score 0, 1, 2, 3 for the placebo, 10mg, 20mg and 40mg groups, respectively. The interaction between ADA and dose was also included. The parameter estimates are shown in Table 4.9. Based on the results from the Cox regression analysis, ADA status does not significant impact RA recurrence (p-value=0.47), but the dose significantly lower the recurrence rates (p-value=0.01). Additionally, the interaction effect between ADA and dose is not statistically significant (p-value=0.89).

4.4.3   Effect of ADA on Longitudinal Outcomes

Longitudinal studies are used to measure changes in endpoints of interest over time and play a key role in epidemiology, clinical research, and therapeutic

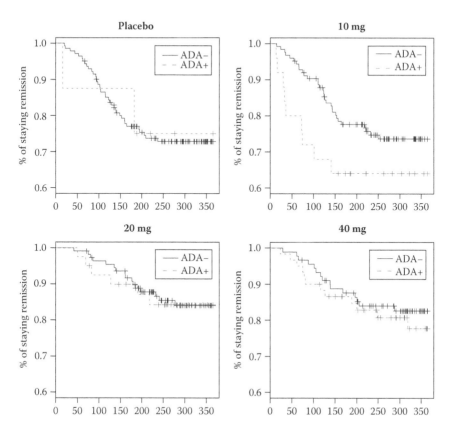

FIGURE 4.3
Kaplan–Meier estimates of % of subjects staying in remission by ADA status
for the four dose groups.

TABLE 4.8
Stratified log-rank test for the effect of ADA on remission after controlling for
dose level

		# of recurrence		
ADA Status	# of subjects	Observed	Expected	T^2_{SLR}
ADA−	467	99	104	1.4
ADA+	133	29	24	

TABLE 4.9
Parameter estimates of the Cox model for RA recurrence

Covariate	β	$\exp(\beta)$	$SE(\beta)$	Z	p-value
ADA status	0.32	1.37	0.44	0.73	0.47
Dose	-0.23	0.79	0.09	-2.44	0.01
ADA-Dose interaction	-0.03	0.97	0.21	-0.13	0.89

evaluation. For example, longitudinal studies are used to characterize normal growth and aging, to assess the effect of risk factors on human health, and to evaluate the effectiveness of treatments. A longitudinal study generates multiple or repeated measurement on each subject. For example, patients with RA may be followed over a period of two years in a clinical trial. The RA symptoms, DAS28 scores and other biomarkers may be collected to monitor disease progression. The repeated measurements are correlated within each subject and require special statistical techniques for valid analysis and inference.

For example, suppose that there are a total of n subjects in the study and the ith subject has n_i observations. Let Y_{ij} denote the random variable for the response and let $\boldsymbol{x}_{ij} = (x_{ij1}, \cdots, x_{ijp})$ denote the vector of p covariates for the jth observation for the ith subject, $j = 1, ..., n_i$. The entire set of observations for the ith subject is denoted as

$$\boldsymbol{Y}_i = \begin{pmatrix} Y_{i1} \\ Y_{i2} \\ \vdots \\ Y_{in_i} \end{pmatrix}, \boldsymbol{x}_i = \begin{pmatrix} \boldsymbol{x}_{i1} \\ \boldsymbol{x}_{i2} \\ \vdots \\ \boldsymbol{x}_{in_i} \end{pmatrix}, \boldsymbol{\mu}_i = \begin{pmatrix} \mu_{i1} \\ \mu_{i2} \\ \vdots \\ \mu_{in_i} \end{pmatrix}, i = 1, ..., n, \quad (4.50)$$

The total number of observations is $N = \sum_{i=1}^{n} n_i$. In a longitudinal clinical trial, each unit is measured on several occasions. Since it is likely that multiple observations for the same individual are correlated or clustered, it is necessary to take the correlation into account. Two types of models, e.g., the marginal model and the mixed-effects model, are commonly used to analyze longitudinal data.

For example, in a longitudinal clinical trial, the efficacy of the mAb under investigation on RA may be investigated. To assess the impact of ADA on efficacy, we would like to estimate the effect of ADA response in the presence of treatment. Let Y_{ij} denote the binary indicator for the presence of RA recurrence and let $\boldsymbol{x}_{ij} = (x_{ij1}, x_{ij2})$ be the bivariate vector of covariates. Here, we assume that x_{ij1} is the indicator of being in the treatment group ($x_{ij1} = 1$) versus in the placebo group ($x_{ij1} = 0$) and x_{ij2} is the indicator of having ADA response.

TABLE 4.10
Common distributions from the exponential family

Distribution	Density or probability function	η	ϕ
Gaussian	$f(y\|\mu,\sigma^2) = \frac{1}{\sqrt{2\pi\sigma^2}}\exp\left(-\frac{(y-\mu)^2}{2\sigma^2}\right), y \in \mathbb{R}$	μ	σ^2
Bernoulli	$f(y\|\pi) = \pi^y(1-\pi)^{1-y}, y \in \{0,1\}.$	$\log(\frac{\pi}{1-\pi})$	1
Poisson	$f(y\|\lambda) = \frac{\lambda^y}{y!}\exp(-\lambda), y \in \{0,1,2,...\}$	$\log(\lambda)$	1
Exponential	$f(y\|\lambda) = \lambda\exp(-\lambda y), y \in \mathbb{R}^+$	$-\lambda$	1

4.4.3.1 Generalized Linear Model

Before we present the statistical models for longitudinal outcomes, we briefly describe the generalized linear models (GLMs) for random variables from the exponential family (Wedderburn (1974); McCullagh and Nelder (1989)). The exponential family represents an important class of probability distributions that share a certain functional form. The distributions from the exponential family include many of the most common distributions, e.g. the Gaussian (normal), exponential, gamma, chi-square, beta, Bernoulli, Poisson, inverse Wishart distributions (Johnson et al. (1994, 1995)). A random variable Y follows a distribution from the exponential family, if the density or probability mass function takes the form

$$f(y|\eta,\phi) = \exp\{\phi^{-1}[\eta y - \psi(\eta)] + c(y,\phi)\} \tag{4.51}$$

with known functions $\psi(\cdot)$ and $c(\cdot,\cdot)$ and natural parameter η and scale parameter ϕ. The mean and variance of the random variable Y are $\mu = E(Y) = \phi'(\eta)$ and $\sigma^2 = \text{Var}(Y) = \phi\psi''(\eta)$, respectively. The density functions of several commonly used distributions are shown in Table 4.10. Among them, the normal distribution with mean μ and variance σ^2 is denoted as $N(\mu,\sigma^2)$.

Suppose that there are n subjects in the study. For the ith subject, the response is denoted by Y_i and the vector of covariates is denote as $\boldsymbol{x}_i = (x_{i1},..,x_{ip})'$, $i = 1,...n$. Let $\mu_i = E(Y_i|\boldsymbol{x}_i)$ be the expectation of Y_i. The GLM (McCulloch and Searle (2004); Dobson and Barnett (2008)) assumes that the response Y_i comes from an exponential-family distribution with density function $f(y|\eta_i,\phi)$ and

$$g^{-1}(\mu_i) = \eta_i = \boldsymbol{x}_i'\boldsymbol{\beta}, \tag{4.52}$$

where $\eta_i = g(\mu_i)$ with the link function $g(\cdot)$ and $\boldsymbol{\beta} = (\beta_1,...,\beta_p)'$ is the vector of regression coefficients. The estimates of $\boldsymbol{\beta}$ are usually obtained using the maximum likelihood method. For independent observations $(y_1,...,y_n)$, the log-likelihood function and the corresponding score equation are

$$L(\boldsymbol{\beta}, \phi) = \frac{1}{\phi} \sum_{i=1}^{n} [y_i \eta_i - \psi(\eta_i)] + \sum_{i1=}^{n} c(y_i, \phi),$$

$$S(\boldsymbol{\beta}) = \sum_{i=1}^{n} \frac{\partial \eta_i}{\partial \boldsymbol{\beta}} [y_i - \psi'(\eta_i)] = \sum_{i=1}^{n} \frac{\partial \mu_i}{\partial \boldsymbol{\beta}} v_i^{-1} [y_i - \mu_i] = 0.$$

where $\mu_i = \psi'(\eta_i)$ and $v_i = \psi''(\eta_i)$. Using simple algebra for derivatives, $\frac{\partial \mu_i}{\partial \boldsymbol{\beta}} = \psi''(\eta_i) \frac{\partial \eta_i}{\partial \boldsymbol{\beta}}$. The estimates of $\boldsymbol{\beta}$ are often obtained numerically, e.g., iteratively reweighted least squares method, Newton–Raphson method or the Fisher scoring method. The corresponding likelihood ratio test, Wald test, and score tests can be derived based on asymptotic theory (Dobson and Barnett (2008)). The commonly used GLMs include the logistic regression model for binary responses and the Poisson regression model for count responses.

4.4.3.2   Marginal Generalized Linear Model

In a marginal model, the marginal regression of the longitudinal or clustered responses is modeled separately from the within-subject correlation. Let $\mu_{ij} = E(y_{ij})$ be the marginal expectation of the response y_{ij}. The marginal expectation is associated with the covariates $\boldsymbol{x}_{ij}$ via a GLM:

$$g(\mu_{ij}) = \boldsymbol{\beta}' \boldsymbol{x}_{ij}, \tag{4.53}$$

where $g(\cdot)$ is the link function. The commonly used link functions for binary response include logit, inverse log-log or probit functions. The marginal variance of Y_{ij} depends on the marginal mean as $\text{Var}(Y_{ij}) = V(\mu_{ij})\phi$, where $V(\cdot)$ is a known variance function and ϕ is an unknown scale parameter. The correlations between Y_{ij} and Y_{ik} is a function of the marginal mean with a possible additional parameter $\boldsymbol{\theta}$, i.e., $\text{Corr}(Y_{ij}, Y_{ik}) = \rho(\mu_{ij}, \mu_{ik}, \boldsymbol{\theta})$, where $\rho(\cdot)$ is a known function.

For the marginal models, the regression coefficients are the primary parameters of interest. In the RA example, $\mu_{ij} = E(Y_{ij}) = \Pr(Y_{ij} = 1)$ is the probability of RA recurrence and the marginal recurrence probability is given by

$$\text{logit}(\mu_{ij}) = \log\left(\frac{\mu_{ij}}{1 - \mu_{ij}}\right) = \beta_0 + \beta_1 x_{ij1} + \beta_2 x_{ij2},$$
$$\text{Var}(Y_{ij}) = \mu_{ij}(1 - \mu_{ij}).$$

We assume that the correlation structure between Y_{ij} and Y_{ik} is specified as $\text{Corr}(Y_{ij}, Y_{ik}) = \rho$, which means homogeneous equal correlations. The transformed regression coefficient $\exp(\beta_1)$ measures the odds ratio of having RA recurrence for the treated group versus the placebo group.

Because the likelihood function for the marginal model is very complicated, it is convenient to estimate β by solving a multivariate quasi-score function (Wedderburn (1974)). This approach is also called the generalized estimating equation (GEE), which was originally developed by Zeger and Liang (1986); Liang and Zeger (1986); Zeger et al. (1988).

$$\boldsymbol{\mu}_i = \begin{pmatrix} \mu_{i1} \\ \mu_{i2} \\ \vdots \\ \mu_{in_i} \end{pmatrix}, i = 1, ..., n, \tag{4.54}$$

The GEE quasi-score function is formulated as

$$\mathbf{S}_{\boldsymbol{\beta}}(\boldsymbol{\beta}, \boldsymbol{\theta}) = \sum_{i=1}^{N} \left(\frac{\partial \boldsymbol{\mu}_i}{\partial \boldsymbol{\beta}} \right)' \text{Var}(\boldsymbol{Y}_i)^{-1} (\boldsymbol{Y}_i - \boldsymbol{\mu}_i) = \mathbf{0}. \tag{4.55}$$

The estimates of the GEE can be obtained using SAS PROC GENMOD or R function *GEE* (Halekoh et al. (2006)).

4.4.3.3 Generalized Linear Mixed Model

Generalized linear mixed model (GLMM) is another popular model for longitudinal or clustered data analysis. In the mixed-effects models, the distribution of responses $\boldsymbol{Y}_i$ involves a subject-specific random effects $\boldsymbol{b}_i$ as

$$f(\boldsymbol{Y}_i, \boldsymbol{b}_i | \boldsymbol{x}_i, \boldsymbol{z}_i, \boldsymbol{\beta}, \boldsymbol{\theta}) = f(\boldsymbol{Y}_i | \boldsymbol{b}_i, \boldsymbol{x}_i, \boldsymbol{\beta}) f(\boldsymbol{b}_i | \boldsymbol{z}_i, \boldsymbol{\theta}). \tag{4.56}$$

where $\boldsymbol{x}_i$ is the vector of covariates for the fixed effects $\boldsymbol{\beta}$, $\boldsymbol{z}_i$ is the subject-specific vector of covariates for the random effects $\boldsymbol{b}_i$ and $\boldsymbol{\theta}$ is the vector of parameter related to random-effects $\boldsymbol{b}_i$.

The unconditional distribution of response is obtained by integrating $\boldsymbol{b}_i$ out of the joint distribution

$$f(\boldsymbol{Y}_i | \boldsymbol{x}_i, \boldsymbol{z}_i, \boldsymbol{\beta}, \boldsymbol{\theta}) = \int f(\boldsymbol{Y}_i | \boldsymbol{b}_i, \boldsymbol{x}_i, \boldsymbol{\beta}) f(\boldsymbol{b}_i | \boldsymbol{z}_i, \boldsymbol{\theta}) \mathrm{d}\boldsymbol{b}_i. \tag{4.57}$$

Let $\mu_{ij}^b = E(Y_{ij} | \boldsymbol{x}_{ij}, \boldsymbol{z}_{ij}, \boldsymbol{b}_i)$ be the conditional expectation of response Y_{ij} given the covariates $\boldsymbol{x}_i$ and random effects $\boldsymbol{b}_i$. The GLMM specifies the conditional expectation μ_{ij}^b as

$$g(\mu_{ij}^b) = \boldsymbol{x}_{ij}\boldsymbol{\beta} + \boldsymbol{z}_{ij}\boldsymbol{b}_i, \tag{4.58}$$

where $g(\cdot)$ is the link function, $\boldsymbol{x}_{ij}$ is the covariate vector for the fixed effects $\boldsymbol{\beta}$ and $\boldsymbol{z}_{ij}$ is the covariate vector for the random effects $\boldsymbol{b}_i$. The term *mixed-effects model* arise from the representation of both fixed and random effects in the same model. The fixed effects $\boldsymbol{\beta}$ represent the covariate effects at the population level and $\boldsymbol{b}_i$ represents the effects at the individual level. The within-subject covariance matrix $\Sigma_i^b(\psi) = \text{Cov}(\boldsymbol{Y}_i | \boldsymbol{x}_i, \boldsymbol{z}_i, \boldsymbol{b}_i, \gamma)$ usually takes a simple structure, where ψ is the vector of parameters for the correlation matrix. For example, the commonly used covariance matrices include the exchangeable covariance $Cov(Y_{ij}, Y_{ik}) = \sigma[\rho + (1 - \rho)\mathbf{I}(j = k)]$ and the AR(1) covariance $Cov(Y_{ij}, Y_{ik}) = \sigma\rho^{|j-k|}$. The distribution of the random-effects $\boldsymbol{b}_i$ is often assumed to be multivariate normal (MVN)

$$\boldsymbol{b}_i | \boldsymbol{x}_i \sim N(0, \Omega). \tag{4.59}$$

For the MVN response with an identity link function, the marginal distribution of $\boldsymbol{Y}_i$ follows

$$\boldsymbol{Y}_i | \boldsymbol{x}_i, \boldsymbol{z}_i \sim MVN(\boldsymbol{x}_i\boldsymbol{\beta}, \boldsymbol{z}_i\Omega\boldsymbol{z}_i' + \Sigma_i^b). \tag{4.60}$$

Using the RA recurrence example, the binary recurrence status Y_{ij} follows a Bernoulli model distribution

$$Y_{ij} \sim \text{Bernoulli}(\mu_{ij}^b), \tag{4.61}$$

where $g(\mu_{ij}^b) = \boldsymbol{x}_{ij}\boldsymbol{\beta} + \boldsymbol{z}_{ij}\boldsymbol{b}_i$. If a logit link function is used, i.e., $g(\mu_{ij}^b) = \log[\mu_{ij}^b/(1 - \mu_{ij}^b)]$, the resulting model is a random-effects logistic model. The effects of treatment x_{ij1} and ADA response x_{ij2} can be formulated as

$$\text{logit}(\mu_{ij}^b) = \beta_0 + \beta_1 x_{ij1} + \beta_2 x_{ij2} + b_i.$$

Using the matrix notation, the GLMM can be specified as

$$g\{E(\boldsymbol{Y}|\boldsymbol{b})\} = \boldsymbol{X}\boldsymbol{\beta} + \boldsymbol{Z}\boldsymbol{b}, \tag{4.62}$$

where $\boldsymbol{X}$ and $\boldsymbol{Z}$ are the design matrices for fixed and random effects, $\boldsymbol{b}$ is the vector of all random effects.

Let $\boldsymbol{\theta} = (\boldsymbol{\theta}_0, \phi)$, where $\boldsymbol{\theta}_0$ includes all unknown parameters in Σ_b. The parameter estimates can be obtained by maximizing the marginal likelihood function

$$
\begin{aligned}
L(\boldsymbol{\beta}, \boldsymbol{\theta}|\boldsymbol{X}, \boldsymbol{Z}, \boldsymbol{Y}) &= \prod_{i=1}^{N} f(\boldsymbol{Y}_i | \boldsymbol{x}_i, \boldsymbol{\beta}, \boldsymbol{\theta}) \\
&= \prod_{i=1}^{N} \int f(\boldsymbol{Y}_i | \boldsymbol{b}_i, \boldsymbol{x}_i, \boldsymbol{\beta}) f(\boldsymbol{b}_i | \boldsymbol{z}_i, \boldsymbol{\theta}) \mathrm{d}\boldsymbol{b}_i \\
&= \prod_{i=1}^{N} \int \left(\prod_{j=1}^{n_i} f(y_{ij} | \boldsymbol{x}_{ij}, \boldsymbol{\beta}, \phi) f(\boldsymbol{b}_i | \boldsymbol{\theta}) \right) \mathrm{d}\boldsymbol{b}_i. \quad (4.63)
\end{aligned}
$$

For the GLMM with multivariate normal random effects where $\boldsymbol{b}_i \sim MVN(0, \Sigma_b)$, the marginal distribution is also a normal distribution. In general, numerical approximation should be used for non-normal outcomes. Different approaches have been used to approximate the likelihood function (4.63).

The estimating equation can be obtained by using a Laplace approximation of the marginal likelihood function(Breslow and Clayton (1993)):

$$L(\boldsymbol{\beta}, \boldsymbol{\theta}) \propto \prod_{i=1}^{n} \int \exp\{Q(\boldsymbol{b}_i)\} d\boldsymbol{b}_i \qquad (4.64)$$

where

$$Q(\boldsymbol{b}_i) = -\frac{1}{\phi} \sum_{j=1}^{n_i} [(y_{ij} - \psi)(\boldsymbol{x}'_{ij}\boldsymbol{\beta} + \boldsymbol{Z}'_{ij}\boldsymbol{b}_i] - \frac{1}{2}\boldsymbol{b}'_i \Sigma_b^{-1} \boldsymbol{b}_i. \qquad (4.65)$$

Let $\hat{\boldsymbol{b}}$ be the value that maximize $Q(\boldsymbol{b})$ and $Q(\boldsymbol{b})$ can be approximated by a second-order Taylor approximation

$$Q(\boldsymbol{b}) \approx Q(\hat{\boldsymbol{b}}) + \frac{1}{2}(\boldsymbol{b} - \hat{b}b)' Q''(\hat{\boldsymbol{b}})(\boldsymbol{b} - \hat{\boldsymbol{b}}). \qquad (4.66)$$

Therefore, the marginal likelihood function can be approximated as

$$L(\boldsymbol{\beta}, \boldsymbol{\theta}) = \prod_{i=1}^{n} \int \exp\{Q(\boldsymbol{b}_i)\} d\boldsymbol{b}_i = \prod_{i=1}^{n} (2\pi)\frac{q}{2} | - Q''(\hat{\boldsymbol{b}}_i)|^{-\frac{1}{2}} \exp\{Q(\hat{\boldsymbol{b}}_i)\}, \quad (4.67)$$

where

$$
\begin{aligned}
-Q''(\boldsymbol{b}_i) &= -\Sigma_b^{-1} + \phi^{-1} \sum_{j=1}^{n_i} \boldsymbol{z}_{ij} \psi''(\boldsymbol{x}'_{ij}\boldsymbol{\beta} + \boldsymbol{z}'_{ij}\boldsymbol{b}_i)\boldsymbol{z}_{ij} \\
&= \Sigma_b^{-1} + \phi^{-1} \boldsymbol{Z}'_i \boldsymbol{V}_i \boldsymbol{Z}_i
\end{aligned}
$$

where $\boldsymbol{V}_i = \mathrm{diag}(\mathrm{Var}(Y_{ij}|\boldsymbol{b}_i))$. The estimates $\hat{\boldsymbol{b}}_i$ depend on the unknown parameters $\boldsymbol{\beta}$ and $\boldsymbol{\theta}$. The approximate MLEs can be obtained by iterating the likelihood function between updating $\hat{\boldsymbol{b}}_i$ and $(\hat{\boldsymbol{\beta}}, \hat{\boldsymbol{\theta}})$. In addition to the Laplace approximation, some alternative estimation methods include the Pseudo-likelihood method based on linearization, penalized quasi-likelihood (PQL) method, adaptive Gaussian quadrature (Pinheiro and Chao (2006)), and the EM algorithm (Booth and Hobert (1999)). The default method in PROC GLIMMIX is the pseudo-likelihood method and the default method in R functions *lme4* and *glmer* is the Laplace approximation method.

4.4.3.4 Generalized Additive Model

A generalized additive model (GAM)(Hastie and Tibshirani (1990)) is a flexible extension of the GLMs with a linear predictor involving a sum of smooth functions of covariates. Let $\boldsymbol{x}_i = (x_{i1}, x_{i2}, ..., x_{ip})$ be the vector of covariates and let Y_i be the response for the ith subject. Suppose y_i is an observed value of Y_i from the exponential-family distribution.

The GAM is specified as

$$g(\mu_i) = \boldsymbol{A}_i \boldsymbol{\theta} + \sum_j L_{ij} \xi_j(x_{ij}), \qquad (4.68)$$

where $g(\cdot)$ is the link function, $\mathbf{A}_i$ is the ith row of a model matrix for any parametric terms, $\xi_j(\cdot)$ is a smooth function of covariate $x_{\cdot p}$. Because the smooth function ξ's are confounded with the intercept term, usually constraints $\sum_i \xi_j(x_{ij}) = 0$ for all j are imposed for the sake of identifiability. The parameter estimates of $\boldsymbol{\beta}$ can be obtained using the penalized likelihood method.

For longitudinal data $(y_{ij}, \boldsymbol{x}_{ij}), i = 1, ..., n, j = 1, ..., n_i$, a generalized additive mixed model (GAMM) takes the form

$$g(\mu_{ij}) = \mathbf{A}_i \boldsymbol{\theta} + \sum_k L_{ik} \xi_k(x_{ik}) + \mathbf{Z}_i b_i, \qquad (4.69)$$

where $\mu_{ij} = E(y_{ij})$, the random effects $\boldsymbol{b}_i \sim N(0, \Sigma_b)$. The estimation of GAM and GAMM has been implemented in various statistical packages, e.g, PROC GAM and R functions *gam* and *gamm*.

GAMs are very important tools for explanatory data analysis. One of the main advantages of the GAMs is that it offers great flexibility for representing the relations between the dependant variable and the covariates. Additionally, GAMs can accommodate many complicated nonlinear model, e.g. growth-curve model or dose-response model. Additive models are not only more parsimonious than the general non-parametric models, but also easier to interpret. For more discussions about the GAM and GAMM, see Hastie and Tibshirani (1990) and Wood (2006).

4.4.3.5   Example

The RA patients were followed up over time and the secondary endpoint DAS28 scores were measured at month 0 (baseline) and months 4, 8, 16, 24, 32, 40, 48, and 56. As multiple measurements were taken of each subject, the correlation among the repeated measurements were taken into account in order to assess the effects of dose level and ADA. Here, we consider two covariates dose level and ADA status.

We assume the expected mean value for DAS28 score is specified as

$$
\begin{aligned}
E(y_{ij}) &= \mu_{ij} \\
&= \beta_0 + \beta_1 I(x_{i1} = 1) + \beta_2 I(x_{i1} = 2) + \beta_2 I(x_{i1} = 3) + \beta_4 t_{ij} \\
&\quad + \beta_5 I(x_{i1} = 1) t_{ij} + \beta_6 I(x_{i1} = 2) t_{ij} + \beta_7 I(x_{i1} = 3) t_{ij} \\
&\quad + \beta_8 x_{i2}, \qquad (4.70)
\end{aligned}
$$

where t_{ij} is the time of measurement, dose level $x_{i1} = 0, 1, 2, 3$ denotes placebo, 10mg, 20mg and 40mg group, respectively and the variable for ADA x_{i2} is binary with $x_{i2} = 1$ for ADA+ subjects and $x_{i2} = 0$ for ADA− subjects. First, we fit a marginal linear model using the R function *geeglm* with an exchangeable correlation matrix. The parameter estimates of the coefficients are shown in Table 4.11. The average difference DAS28 scores between the three treatment groups and the placebo group ranged between 0.851 and 0.934

TABLE 4.11

Parameter estimates of the marginal linear model for DAS28 from GEE

Variable	Estimate	Std.err	Wald χ^2	p-value
Intercept	6.150	0.120	2625.259	<0.001
Dose group x_{i1}				
10 mg	-0.851	0.153	30.863	<0.001
20 mg	-0.934	0.153	37.114	<0.001
40 mg	-0.863	0.156	30.516	<0.001
Time t_{ij}	-0.005	0.003	2.685	0.101
Time*Dose $(x_{i1} * t_{ij})$				
Time*$I(x_{i1} = 1)$	-0.028	0.004	51.914	<0.001
Time*$I(x_{i1} = 2)$	-0.035	0.004	97.798	<0.001
Time*$I(x_{i1} = 3)$	-0.059	0.004	277.137	<0.001
ADA (x_{i2})	0.236	0.105	5.080	0.024

(all p-values< 0.001). The regression coefficient for time was -0.005, which was the monthly decrease of the DAS28 score for the placebo group. This means that the DAS28 score remained roughly unchanged for the placebo group, while the DAS28 scores for the three treated groups decreased significantly over time. The difference of DAS28 due to ADA response was 0.236 with p-value= 0.024. This means that subjects with detectable ADA have higher DAS28 score relative to the placebo group. The estimate of correlation among repeated measurements was 0.418 with standard error 0.0235. Therefore, the multiple measurements of DAS28 for the same subjects are highly correlated.

We also fit a linear mixed-effects model with a random intercept to the DAS28 score:

$$E(y_{ij}|b_i) = \mu_{ij} + b_i \qquad (4.71)$$

where μ_{ij} is specified in equation (4.70). The parameter estimates from the linear mixed-effects model are shown in Table 4.12. The estimates from the random-intercept model are identical to those from the marginal linear model, while the estimates from the random-effects have slightly smaller standard error. In general, the estimates from the linear mixed-effects model and the marginal linear model may be slightly different.

We also fit a GAMM to estimate the trajectory of DAS28 (Figure 4.4). In each sub-figure, the trajectories of the DAS28 for the ADA+ and ADA− subjects are plotted. The additive model is useful to depict the nonlinear trajectory of response variables over time. As shown in Figure 4.4, the DAS28 scores of the placebo group remained unchanged over time. The DAS28 scores of each of the three treatment groups decreased until month 30, then leveled off. Subjects treated with the highest dose (40mg) had the largest drop in DAS28. This indicates that the reduction of DAS28 was dose-dependent.

TABLE 4.12

Parameter estimates of the random-intercept model

Variable	Estimate	Std. Error	t value	p-value
Intercept	6.150	0.102	60.332	<0.001
Dose group x_{i1}				
10mg	-0.851	0.145	-5.882	<0.001
20mg	-0.934	0.146	-6.405	<0.001
40mg	-0.863	0.148	-5.823	<0.001
Time (t_{ij})	-0.005	0.002	-1.891	0.059
Time*Dose $(x_{i1} * t_{ij})$				
Time*$I(x_{i1} = 1)$	-0.028	0.004	-7.904	<0.001
Time*$I(x_{i1} = 2)$	-0.035	0.003	-10.057	<0.001
Time*$I(x_{i1} = 3)$	-0.059	0.003	-17.087	<0.001
ADA (x_{i2})	0.236	0.107	2.192	0.029

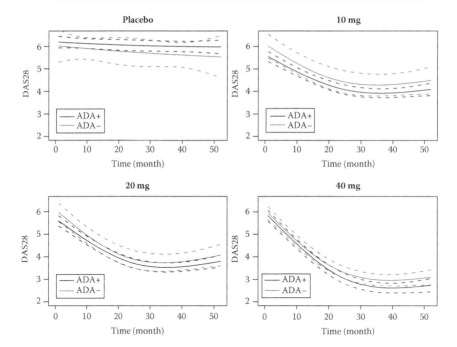

FIGURE 4.4

Trajectory of DAS28 by ADA status for the four treatment groups.

4.5 Effect of ADA on AEs

During drug clinical development and post-licensure, AE monitoring is crucial for protecting patient safety. As defined in 21 CFR 312.32(a), pre-licensure, and 21 CFR 314.80, post licensure, an AE is defined as "any untoward medical occurrence associated with the use of a drug in humans, whether or not considered drug related" throughout product life cycle according to the Code of Federal Regulations (21 CFR 312.32) and ICH E6 "Guideline for Good Clinical Practice". An AE can be any unfavorable sign, symptom or disease; it can be any abnormal laboratory, imaging, ECG test result. A serious AE (SAE) refers to the serious event like death, a life-threatening reaction, hospitalization or prolongation of existing hospitalization among other conditions (21 CFR 314.80).

In the drug safety data analysis, one important goal is to identify increased risk, and/or frequency of an AE in the clinical trial. It is equally important to detect treatment-emergent AE as early as possible. But the signal of AEs should also be carefully diagnosed, since the cost of false alarm is expensive and lengthens the drug approval process.

Existing statistical methodology to evaluate the efficacy of a study drug in clinical trials is well-developed. However, the research on the safety profiles, including AE data, is very limited. In most randomized clinical trial, safety profiles are predominantly restricted to exploratory analysis where AEs are tabulated by type, severity(grade), body system and incidence. Recently, regulatory agencies and the pharmaceutical industry have realized the importance of using rigorous statistical analysis on AE data (O'Neill (1995); Chuang-Stein and Mohberg (1993); Chuang-Stein (1998); Chuang-Stein et al. (2001)). The FDA published a series of guidances on how to conduct a clinical safety review and to prepare a report of a new drug application (FDA (1996)) and on how to assess and mitigate safety issues in development. Various statistical techniques have been described to analyze safety data in clinical trials (Southworth (2008); Cao and He (2011)). Typically, the incidence rates of AEs are very low, the statistical method for AE should deal with the challenges of rare event and often zero counts. Here, we are interested in the impact of ADAs on the AEs, after controlling for the effect of treatment.

4.5.1 Statistical Methods for AEs

To assess the effect of ADA on AEs, the AE analysis should adjust for exposure of drugs or dose level. The AEs are often summarized in contingency tables. chi-square test and Fisher's exact test are two most popular approaches. The chi-square test is an asymptotic test based on large sample size. A general rule of thumb is for the expected cell counts to be at least 5, based on a theorem assuming normal approximation of binomial proportion at $np \geq 5$ and $n(1-p) \geq 5$. If any of the cells has expected count less than 5, a Chi-square test will be inappropriate and the Fisher's exact test is the preferred method.

Suppose that we want to compare the AE response probabilities between the ADA+ and ADA− groups. The heterogeneity between study subjects is characterized using stratified factors and a stratified method should be used. Before one can use the stratified tests for multiple 2×2 tables, the assumptions of common ORs or RRs across different strata should be assessed. For testing the common odds ratio assumption, the statistical methods described in Section 4.4.1.1 can be used. If the assumptions of common odds ratios or risk ratios is not satisfied, robust tests that does not require homogeneity of the ORs and RRs have been used. Cochran (1954b) and Mantel and Haenszel (1959) developed an asymptotic test to compare the AE response rates between two groups without the assumption of common OR and RR. Jung (2014) provided sample size calculation for stratified Fisher's exact test. Jung (2014) also showed that the CMH test may not be able to control the type I error rate accurately when the cell counts are small. The one-sided p-value by the stratified Fisher's exact test is much larger than that by CMH possibly because very small count numbers across the strata may lead to a biased p-value for the asymptotic CMH test. The stratified Fisher's exact test can be used to test the effect of ADA on AEs.

Suppose that there are J strata, defined by dose level and/or other covariates and there are K types of AEs. For the kth AE type, the 2×2 table of ADA and AE frequency data for the jth stratum are summarized in Table 4.13. Let N_j denote the total number of subjects in the jth stratum. Among the N_j subjects, m_{j1} are ADA+ and m_{j2} are ADA−, respectively.

Let $d_k, k = 1, ..., K$ be the level for the kth dose group. The data can be stratified in K 2×2 tables as follows:

TABLE 4.13
The 2×2 table of AE and ADA reaction in the jth dose group for the kth AE

	AE +	AE −	
ADA +	$s_{j1}^{(k)}$	$s_{j2}^{(k)}$	m_{j1}
ADA −	$n_{j1}^{(k)} - s_{j1}^{(k)}$	$n_{j2}^{(k)} - s_{j2}^{(k)}$	m_{j2}
All	$n_{j1}^{(k)}$	$n_{j2}^{(k)}$	N_j

For the jth stratum group, the kth type AE rate is $s_{j1}^{(k)}/m_{j1}$ for the ADA+ group and $s_{j1}^{(k)}/m_{j2}$ for the ADA− group. Let $p_1^{(k)} = P(\text{Type } k \text{ AE} = +|\text{ADA}+)$ and $p_2^{(k)} = P(\text{Type } k \text{ AE} = +|\text{ADA}-)$ be the probabilities of kth type AE in the jth group. Let $\theta_j^{(k)} = \frac{p_1^{(k)}/(1-p_1^{(k)})}{p_2^{(k)}/(1-p_2^{(k)})}$ be the odd ratio of having ADA on the kth type AE in stratum j. To test whether the ADA response has an impact on the kth type AE rate, the null and alternative hypotheses

are
$$H_0 : \theta_1^{(k)} = \cdots = \theta_J^{(k)} = 1$$

versus
$$H_1 : \theta_j^{(k)} > 1 \text{ for some } j = 1, ..., J. \tag{4.72}$$

The null hypothesis will be rejected in favor of the alternative hypothesis if $S^{(k)} = \sum_{j=1}^{J} s_{j1}^{(k)}$ is sufficiently large. The p-value of the test can be obtained from the Fisher's exact test, which is based on the hypergeometric distribution.

The Fisher's exact test may be too conservative due to the fact that the number of events are discrete. In contrast, the asymptotic Chi-square tests, like the CMH test, can be liberal as well as conservative for a small sample size or sparse data. When the effect size is so large that the required sample size is small, say, about $N = 70$ or smaller, the exact test needs about 20% to 30% larger sample size than CMH test.

4.5.2 Controlling False Discovery Rate

The AEs in clinical trials are routinely classified into different categories. Statistical tests can be used to compare the AE rates between the ADA+ and ADA− groups after controlling for other confounding factors. The p-values are calculated and reported for each body system. If we simply interpret a p-value less than 0.05 as statistical significance, there is a potential for an increase in false positives. Excess false positive findings can lead to unnecessary false alarm of the safety profile of a safe drug or vaccine. This is an issue of multiplicity because multiple AE types are under consideration simultaneously (Yu et al. (2005)).

Let $\mathbb{H} = \{H_0^{(1)}, ..., H_0^{(K)}\}$ denote a family of K hypotheses. The family-wise error rate (FWER) is defined as the probability that any true hypothesis in the set $\mathbb{H}$ is rejected. Multiple testing procedures aim to control the family-wise error rate such that the FWER is no greater than the pre-specified level α. Benjamini and Hochberg (1995) argued that controlling the FWER is often too conservative and suggested controlling the FDA as a more practical alternative. FDR can be best described by breaking down the K hypotheses in the family $\mathbb{H}$.

TABLE 4.14
The 2×2 table of testing the effect of ADA on all types of AE

	H_0 is not rejected	H_0 is rejected	
H_0 is true	K_{11}	K_{12}	$K_{1\cdot}$
H_0 is false	K_{21}	K_{22}	$K_{2\cdot}$
All	$K_{\cdot 1}$	$K_{\cdot 2}$	K

The FDR is defined as the expected proportion of rejected hypotheses which are incorrectly rejected, $E(K_{12}/K)$. In this application we are considering the K hypotheses $\{H_0^{(1)}, ..., H_0^{(K)}\}$ based on the corresponding p-values, $p_1, p_2, \ldots, p_K$. Let $p_{(1)}, ..., p_{(K)}$ be the ordered p-values. The FDR procedure rejects hypotheses $H_0^{(1)}, ..., H_0^{(k)}$ when

$$k = \max\{l : p_{(l)} \leq \alpha(l/K)\}. \tag{4.73}$$

Benjamini and Hochberg (1995) showed that when all hypotheses are independent this procedure controls the FDR at level $K_1./K\alpha$. The FDR procedure is generally more powerful than the FWER controlling procedures. This property is highly desirable when testing hypotheses regarding AEs. The FDR-adjusted procedure (Benjamini and Hochberg (1995)) can be implemented using the adjusted p-values:

$$\tilde{p}_{(K)} = p_{(K)}$$
$$\tilde{p}_{(l)} = \min\left\{\tilde{p}_{(l+1)}, \frac{K}{l}p_{(l)}\right\} \text{ for } l \leq K - 1.$$

Mehrotra and Heyse (2004) proposed a double FDR approach for flagging AEs. This procedure is appropriate for AEs that were included as part of the overall patient safety report in a clinical trial. This procedure first groups the AEs into pre-defined subsets. These groups may be determined by body systems or other characteristics, e.g., physical disability or cognitive disability, when appropriately based on the underlying mechanism of action for the experimental drug. As an illustration, Mehrotra and Heyse (2004) classified AEs into s categories. For the ith category, there are k_i types of AEs.

The two-step FDR procedure (Mehrotra and Heyse (2004)) for examining the effect of ADA on AEs can be described as following:

1. Calculate the test p-value p_{ij} for comparing two groups, i.e., ADA+ and ADA− groups, for the jth AE in the ith AE category. The test can be any proper statistical test, e.g., the stratified Fisher's exact test in Section 4.5.1.

2. Among the AEs under study, identify the event and AE category that yield statistical significance after adjusting for multiplicity using the double FDR approach.

The double FDR procedure uses $p_i^* = \min(p_{i1}, p_{i2}, \ldots, p_{ik_1})$ as the most significant p-value for the ith AE category. The first level of adjustment applies the FDR procedure to the p-values $\{p_1^*, \ldots, p_s^*\}$. The second level of FDR adjustment is applied to the p-values $\{p_{i1}, p_{i2}, \ldots, p_{ik_1}\}$ within the ith AE category. Let $\tilde{p}_i^*$ and $\tilde{p}_{ij}$ be the adjusted p-values from the two-step adjustments. The AE $AE(i, j)$ for the ith AE category and jth type AE is considered to be significantly different if $\tilde{p}_i^* < \alpha_1$ and $\tilde{p}_{ij} \leq \alpha_2$ for the pre-specified values of α_1 and α_2. Mehrotra and Heyse (2004) also considered how to set the appropriate values for α_1 and α_2 using bootstrap resampling. Recently, Mehrotra and

Adewale (2012) proposed a method for flagging clinical AEs, which reduces FDR, but without compromising the power for detecting true signals.

4.5.3 Bayesian Hierarchical Model

As an alternative to frequentist approaches that adjusts for multiplicity, Berry and Berry (2004) proposed a three-level Bayesian hierarchical mixture model for the analysis of AEs to account for the multiplicity issue. To determine whether the treatment raises the level of AE incidence relative to the control group, they used a logistic model that incorporates the information of treatment option, body system, and AE type. Note that the number of AEs are usually rare (DuMouchel (2012)), fitting a logistic model for rare counts may be numerically unstable or lead to unreliable estimates. The proposed hierarchical model tempers extreme results that may occur due to the rarity of many events and borrow strength across correlated events within the same disease category. Xia et al. (2011) considered a mixture distribution and a log-linear model for the AE. This model is appropriate especially when the numbers for most AEs are zero.

Due to the difficulty of implementation, the Bayesian hierarchical model (Berry and Berry (2004)) has not been widely adopted. To fill the gap, Xia et al. (2011) developed WinBUGS code to fit the Bayesian hierarchical model and its extension. Zink (2013) provided SAS code for the hierarchical modeling and introduced a freely available JMP add-in to assess Markov chain Monte Carlo (MCMC) diagnostics, generate forest plots of equal-tailed and highest posterior density (HPD) credible intervals, and calculate univariate and multivariate posterior probabilities. Here, we describe the extension that can be used to assess the effect of ADA on AEs.

Suppose there are C classes of AEs, which are often grouped by MedDRA system organ class (SOC). Within AE class c, there are K_c events. Here we consider an extension of the hierarchical logistic regression model (Berry and Berry (2004)) to estimate the effect of ADA on AEs. Let $\boldsymbol{x} = (x_1, x_2)$ be the vector of treatment group and ADA status. Assume that both x_1 and x_2 are binary variables. Let $Y_{ck}(\boldsymbol{x})$ be the number of subjects with event k in the cth SOC for the group of with $N_{\boldsymbol{x}}$ subjects. Assume $Y_{ck}(x) \sim \text{Poisson}(N_x p_{ck}(x))$. The response probability of AE can be modeled using a logistic model

$$\log(p_{ck}(\boldsymbol{x})) = \beta_{ck}^{(0)} + \beta_{ck}^{(1)} x_1 + \beta_{ck}^{(2)} x_2 \tag{4.74}$$

The effect of ADA on AE is measured by $\theta_{ck} = \exp(\beta_{ck}^{(2)})$, which is the odds ratio for the ADA effect of event k in system organ class c.

To complete the specification of the Bayesian model, the priors are specified as follows. The stage-1 priors of the parameters are

$$\beta_{ck}^{(j)} \sim N(\mu_c^{(j)}, (\sigma_c^{(j)})^2), j = 0, 1, 2. \tag{4.75}$$

The stage 2 priors for the class-specific AE are

$$\mu_c^{(j)} \sim N(\mu_j, \tau_j^2), (\sigma_c^{(j)})^2 \sim IG(A_j, B_j), j = 0, 1, 2; c = 1, ..., C. \qquad (4.76)$$

The stage-3 priors for the overall mean μ_{j0} and variance τ_{j0}^2 are

$$\mu_j \sim N(\mu_j^*, \tau_j^{*2}), \tau_j^2 \sim IG(A_j^*, B_j^*), j = 0, 1, 2. \qquad (4.77)$$

The hyper-parameters $\{A_j, B_j, \mu_j^*, \tau_j^{*2}, A_j^*, B_j^*, j = 0, 1, 2\}$ are assumed to be fixed. Following Xia et al. (2011), we set $\mu_j^* = 0, A_j = A_j^* = 3, B_j = B_j^* = 1, \tau_j^{*2} = 10$.

Rationale for assumed priors and constants are provided in Berry and Berry (2004) and Xia et al. (2011), though sensitivity analyses should be used to examine the robustness of positive findings to alternate assumptions. Model fit can be assessed using the deviance information criterion, which is obtained through the DIC option in the PROC MCMC statement.

4.5.4 Example

Biologics, either alone or along with other RA medications, are increasingly being used to treat moderate to severe RA that has not responded adequately to other treatments. A clear understanding of the common and serious side-effects are very important for proper use of the biologics for the treatment of RA.

The numbers of AEs by event type, treatment group and ADA status are shown in Table 4.15. For illustration, the subjects were divided into two strata according to the dose levels, i.e., $\leq$ 10mg and $>$ 10mg, i.e., the $\leq$ 10 mg group includes the placebo and the 10 mg dose group and the $>$ 10 mg group includes the 20 and 40 mg groups. The effect of ADA response on the AE rate after controlling for the dose level was tested using Zelen's test (Zelen (1971)) for common odds ratio. The unadjusted p-values for each event type are shown in the second to the last column of Table 4.15. Based on the results of the Zelen's test, the ADA+ patients had significantly higher rates of upper respiratory infection and urinary tract infection. Here, we applied the double FDR procedure to evaluate the effects of ADA on AEs. The FDR rate was calculated for the p-values $\{P_{i1}, P_{i2}, ..., P_{ik_i}\}$ for each category of side effects. For example, for upper respiratory infection, the unadjusted p-value was 0.0019 and the FDR was 0.011 among the mild side effects. The minimum p-values for the four side-effects categories were 0.0019, 0.5518, 1.0000 and 0.5969. When the FDR procedure was applied to the minimum p-values, the FDR for the four side effect categories were 0.0076, 0.7959, 1.0000 and 0.7959. By setting $\alpha_1 = \alpha_2 = 0.05$, $\tilde{P}_{ij} = 0.011 < 0.05$ and $\tilde{P}_i^* = 0.0076 < 0.05$. Therefore, the ADA+ subjects had significantly higher upper respiratory infection than those without ADA reaction and there were no significant differences in other AEs.

TABLE 4.15
AEs by event type, treatment group and ADA status

Event type	Description	Dose ≤ 10 mg			Dose > 10 mg				
		Total	ADA+	ADA−	Total	ADA+	ADA−	p-value	FDR
Mild side effects	Injection site reactions	33	7	26	42	8	34	0.2624	0.456
	Headache	15	3	12	20	4	16	0.3733	0.456
	Diarrhea	8	2	6	11	2	9	0.4558	0.456
	Nausea	11	2	9	15	3	12	0.4313	0.456
	Upper respiratory infection	16	10	6	20	13	7	0.0019	0.011
	Urinary tract infection	8	5	3	9	6	3	0.0369	0.111
Serious infections	Pneumonia	8	2	6	4	1	3	0.5518	1.000
	Nasopharyngitis	3	1	2	6	1	5	0.5611	1.000
	Gastroenteritis	2	0	2	0	0	0	1.0000	1.000
	Arthritis, bacterial	2	0	2	3	1	2	0.8020	1.000
	Chest wall abscess	1	0	1	4	1	3	0.8905	1.000
	Staphylococcal bursitis	2	0	2	4	1	3	0.8020	1.000
Malignancies	Squamous cell skin carcinoma	4	1	3	0	0	0	1.0000	1.000
	Diffuse large B cell lymphoma	2	0	2	0	0	0	1.0000	1.000
	Prostate cancer	4	1	3	1	0	1	1.0000	1.000
	Squamous cell lung carcinoma	2	0	2	0	0	0	1.0000	1.000
	Basal cell carcinoma	0	0	0	4	1	3	1.0000	1.000
Autoimmune events	Psoriasis	6	1	5	4	1	3	0.6134	1.000
	Erythema nodosum	4	1	3	2	0	2	1.0000	1.000
	Leukocytoclastic vasculitis	2	0	2	0	0	0	1.0000	1.000
	Raynaud's phenomenon	4	1	3	4	1	3	0.5969	1.000
	Cutaneous lymphocytic vasculitis	2	0	2	1	0	1	1.0000	1.000
	Episcleritis	2	0	2	0	0	0	1.0000	1.000

4.5.5 Concluding Remarks

Although statistical methods are extremely useful for detecting safety signals, we must be aware that most pre-marketing clinical trials are designed to demonstrate efficacy. Because these trials are usually limited in sample size and study duration and exclude high-risk populations, they have limited power to detect rare but potentially serious AEs. Therefore, post-market surveillance data would be an important tool for assessing the safety of a biologic and its immunogenicity.

4.6 Relationship between ADA and Pharmacokinetics

Pharmacokinetics (PK), sometimes described as what the body does to a drug, refers to the movement of drug into, through, and out of the body. PK provides a mathematical basis to quantify the absorption, distribution, metabolism and excretion of a drug. Therefore, the PK processes are often referred to as ADME. A fundamental understanding of these parameters is required to design an appropriate drug regimen for a patient.

The effectiveness of a dosage regimen is determined in part by the concentration of the drug in the body. Commonly used endpoints in PK analysis include area under the blood concentration-time curve (AUC), clearance, maximum blood concentration ($C_{\max}$), time to reach maximum blood concentration ($T_{\max}$), trough blood concentration ($C_{\min}$), volume of distribution at steady state and half-life ($t_{\frac{1}{2}}$).

Population PK studies the sources and correlates of variability in drug concentrations among individuals who are the target patient population receiving clinically relevant doses of the drug. Certain patient demographical, physiological, pathophysiological, and therapeutic features can alter dose-concentration relationships. For example, steady-state concentrations of drugs eliminated mostly by the kidney are usually greater in patients suffering from renal failure than they are in patients with normal renal function who receive the same drug dosage. Population PK studies seek to identify the measurable factors that cause changes in the dose-concentration relationship and the extent of these changes so that, if such changes are associated with clinically significant shifts in the therapeutic index, the dosage can be appropriately modified.

In traditional PK analysis, subjects are usually healthy volunteers or patients with the disease indication that have been carefully screened to minimize inter-individual variability. As mentioned previously, inter-individual variability is minimized through complex study designs and control schemes such as restrictive inclusion/exclusion criteria.In contrast to traditional PK, the population PK approach encompasses some or all of the following features. Accurate measurement and modeling of PK/PD profile of biological products are necessary to make decisions on proper exposure in preclinical toxicology studies, to select first-time-in-human starting doses for single and multiple dosing regimens to determine the efficacious dose for last-phase clinical trials (Agoram (2009)). As described in previous chapters, administration of biologics can induce undesirable ADA, which may have an impact on the PK/PD characteristics. ADA may increase or decrease the clearance of drug, thus alter the PK and PD profiles. Enhancement of the drug clearance may reduce drug exposure leading to reduced drug efficacy. On the other hand, a reduction in clearance may result in sustained bioavailability, which could lead to increased toxicity and/or efficacy. For example, the normal half-life of IgGs is approximately two to three weeks. However, in ADA+ patients, the clearance of an IgG mAbs may be faster as compared to ADA- subjects due to ADA-mAb immune complex formation (Wolbink et al. (2009)). For example, Figure 4.5 shows the blood concentrations of a drug over time in ADA+ and ADA- patients. We see that the ADA+ patients have faster clearance rates as compared to ADA- patients. Because of the potential effect of ADAs on PK and PD, statistical analyses can be useful in determining the clinical relevance of ADAs on PK/PD of the therapeutic.

Nonlinear regression models are widely used in PK and PD analysis, e.g., population PK and PD modeling, or dose-response characterization and dose selection. Such models are often nonlinear mixed-effects models. The population PK modeling can be used to assess the effects of covariates, e.g., age, weight, concomitant medications, comorbidity on PK or PD, to define optimal dosing regimen that will maximize efficacy and/or safety, to provide guidance for choosing dosing regimens for pivotal studies and labeling, and for future studies, e.g., drug-drug interaction. In addition, by including the random-effects model in the nonlinear models, one can estimate both intra-patient and inter-patient variability.

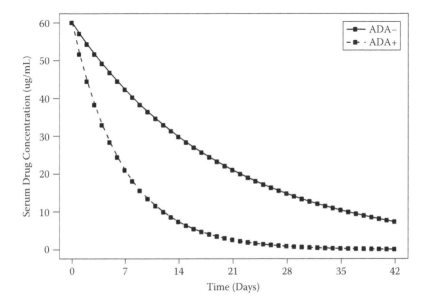

FIGURE 4.5
Concentration of drug as a function of time.

4.6.1 Nonlinear Mixed-Effects Models

We consider a first-order one-compartment model for the blood concentration over time:

$$C(t) = \frac{D}{V} \exp\left(-\frac{CL}{V}t\right). \tag{4.78}$$

The parameter V is the volume of distribution, a larger number means that the drug is distributed to a greater extent into the rest of the body from the circulating blood. The parameter CL denotes the drug clearance (L/hour), which is calculated as

$$CL = \text{Dose} \times F/\text{AUC} \tag{4.79}$$

where Dose is the dose level, F is the bioavailability, AUC is the area under the concentration-time curve. Figure 4.5 shows a typical trajectory of blood concentration of drug overtime after administration of one dose.

Let y_{ij} be the jth response at time t_{ij} for the ith subject. We only consider time-independent covariates $x_i = (x_{i1}, x_{i2})$ where x_{i1} is the treatment group and x_{i2} is the ADA status. The fixed-effects are used to characterize the population mean value of the PK/PD parameters and the variability among the individuals are modeled by the random effects. A mixed-effects model with additive errors can be written as

$$y_{ij} = C(t_{ij}|x_i) = \frac{D_i}{V_i} \exp\left(-t_{ij}\frac{CL_i}{V_i}\right) + \epsilon_{ij} \tag{4.80}$$

where $\epsilon_{ij} \sim N(0, \sigma_\epsilon^2)$ are i.i.d random errors, CL_i is the clearance and V_i is the volume of distribution for the ith subject. The subject-specific parameters can be modeled as

$$\log(CL_i) = \mu_1 + \beta_1 x_{i1} + \beta_2 x_{i2} + b_{i1},$$
$$\log(V_i) = \mu_2 + b_{i2},$$

where the random-effects $b_i = (b_{i1}, b_{i2})' \sim N(\mathbf{0}, \Sigma_b)$ with mean 0 and variance-covariance matrix Σ_b. The parameter estimates can be obtained using SAS PROC NLMIXED.

4.6.2 Pharmacokinetics Model for Multiple Doses

When multiple doses are administrated, the mean function for the accumulating dose need to be constructed recursively. We assume that the drug is given every 24 hours, i.e., at hours 0, 24, 48, etc., with the same dose amount at each dosing time. Let $C(t)$ denote the drug concentration at time t after a single dose. When $0 \le t < 24$ hours, the mean concentration is $C(t)$ as only the first dose is in effect. When $24 \le t < 48$ hours, the predicted concentration is $C(t) + C(t - 24)$ as both doses are in effect. The predicted concentrations at other time points can be similarly derived. Figure 4.6 illustrates the drug concentration over time after administration of multiple doses.

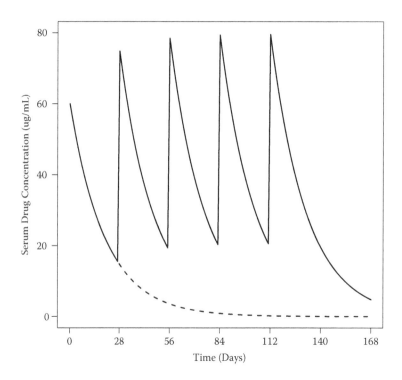

FIGURE 4.6
Drug concentration over time after administration of multiple doses.

Su et al. (2009) described a nonlinear mixed-effects compartmental model for multiple doses. We briefly describe the model with the goal of examining the effect of ADA on PK parameters. Assume that a patient individual receives L doses at time $t_1, t_2, ..., t_L$. Denote the dose amount at time t_i as D_i and define the dosing intervals as $\Delta_i = t_{i+1} - t_i$ for $i = 1, ..., L$. We assume a simple first-order compartment model (4.78) for a single dose. Let $t_0 = 0$. The drug concentration at time t after multiple doses can be derived as

$$C(t|CL, V) = \sum_{j=1}^{m} \frac{D_j}{V} \exp\left(-\frac{CL}{V}(t - t_j)\right), \qquad (4.81)$$

for $t_m < t \leq t_{m+1}$.

In the context of nonlinear mixed effects models (Davidian and Giltinan (1995)), PK parameters such as absorption rate, clearance (CL) and volume of distribution (V) are individual specific. We assume that they come from a common distribution, e.g, a lognormal distribution.

Therefore, we adopt the parameterization of CL and V with independent lognormal distributions for inter-individual variability and an additive error structure for within-subject variability. Let CL_i and V_i be subject i's clearance and volume of distribution respectively. Like the PK model after the administration of one dose, we assume that $(\log(CL), \log(V))$ are bivariate random effects. For each individual, let y_{ij} and C_{ij} be the observed and expected concentration at time t_{ij}, respectively. The

$$
\begin{aligned}
y_{ij} &= C_{ij} + \epsilon_{ij} = C(t_{ij}|CL_i, V_i) + \epsilon_{ij}, \epsilon_{ij} \overset{iid}{\sim} N(0, \sigma^2), \\
\log(CL_i) &= \mu_1 + \beta_1 x_{i1} + \beta_2 x_{i2} + b_{i1}, \\
\log(V_i) &= \mu_2 + b_{i2},
\end{aligned}
$$

where the random-effects $\boldsymbol{b}_i = (b_{i1}, b_{i2})' \sim N(\mathbf{0}, \Sigma_b)$ with mean 0 and variance-covariance matrix Σ_b. By conditioning on individual specific PK parameters, the observed drug concentrations y_{ij}'s are allowed to vary around the expected mean concentration C_{ij} so that C_{ij} can be interpreted as the conditional mean or median concentration, depending on the inter-subject error structure.

4.7 Statistical Analysis ADA Onset and Duration

4.7.1 Modeling ADA Onset Times

Onset of ADA refers to the time between the initial administration of the biologic drug and the first instance of treatment-induced ADA (Shankar et al. (2014)). ADA onset time may be right censored if there is no ADA reaction at the end of the follow-up period. For right-censored data, standard non-parametric and semiparametric methods include the Kaplan–Meier estimates for the survival function, the log-rank test for comparing survival functions between two groups and the Cox model for assessing the effects of covariates. Parametric models, e.g., the AFT models, are often used, too.

ADA onset times, similar to the general disease onset times, are usually interval-censored in longitudinal studies because the ADA status of the subjects is assessed only periodically. For example, an individual who is ADA negative at week 4 may present positive ADA response at week 8. The actually ADA onset time is not directly observed, but known to be between week 4 and 8. Therefore, the actual event times are not exactly identified but is known to take place within a certain interval. Common methods for dealing with interval-censored data are midpoint imputation and right imputation. However, these methods may introduce biases of the parameter estimation. Here, we describe several common methods for the analysis of interval-censored data, which can be applied to ADA onset times.

Regardless of the latent event time, the interval-censored event time T of a subject is only observed to lie in the interval $(L, R]$, i.e., after the last assessment with a negative identification of the event and at or before the first positive assessment. If there is no positive assessment at the end of the observation period, the failure time T is considered to be right-censored at the latest assessment time L and $R = \infty$. Parametric and nonparametric likelihood estimates of the survival function for interval-censored data can be obtained using SAS PROC LIFEREG. Variance estimates are computed by inverting the negative of the Hessian matrix of the likelihood functions.

4.7.1.1 Hypothesis Testing for Interval-Censored Data

Consider a sample of n subjects from a homogeneous population with survival function $S(t)$. Let T_i denote the survival time of interest for subject $i, i = 1, ..., n$, and let (L_i, R_i) be the interval for which T_i is located. The likelihood function for the set of observed intervals $(L_i, R_i], i = 1, ..., n\}$ is

$$L = \prod_{i=1}^{n} \{S(L_i) - S(R_i)\}. \tag{4.82}$$

For the observed interval-censored data $(L_i, R_i], i = 1, ..., n\}$, a set of nonoverlapping intervals $\{(l_1, r_1], ..., (l_m, r_m]\}$ is generated over which the survival function can be estimated. The nonparametric maximum likelihood estimator (NPMLE) of $S(t)$ is a decreasing function on the nonoverlapping intervals $\{(l_1, r_1], ..., (l_m, r_m]\}$, so the jump probabilities can be estimated only on these intervals (Peto (1973); Turnbull (1976)). The survival curve is assumed to be constant everywhere except these intervals. Assuming the censoring mechanism is independent of the failure time distribution, the likelihood of the data $\{T_i \in (L_i, R_i], i = 1, ..., n\}$ can be constructed from the pseudoparameters $\{\theta_j = P(l_j < T \le r_j), j = 1, ..., m\}$. The vector parameter $\boldsymbol{\theta} = (\theta_1, ..., \theta_m)$ can be estimated by maximizing the likelihood $L(\boldsymbol{\theta})$ under the constraint

$\sum_{j=1}^{m} \theta_j = 1,$

$$L(\boldsymbol{\theta}) = \prod_{i=1}^{n} \sum_{j=1}^{m} I[(l_j, r_j) \subset (L_i, R_i)]\theta_j. \tag{4.83}$$

The NPMLE of $S(t)$ based on the MLEs $\{\hat{\theta}_1, ..., \hat{\theta}_m\}$ is given by

$$\hat{S}(t) = \begin{cases} 1 & t < l_1 \\ \sum_{k=j+1}^{m} \theta_k & r_j \leq t \leq l_{j+1} \\ 0 & t \geq r_m \end{cases}. \tag{4.84}$$

Gentleman and Geyer (1994) introduced a method to ensure that the solution is a global maximum. Even with a moderate number of parameters, convergence of the EM algorithm is very slow. The iterative convex minorant (ICM) algorithm (Groeneboom et al. (2008)) and the EM iterative convex minorant algorithm (EM-ICM) (Wellner and Zhan (1997)) are much more efficient methods for computing the nonparametric maximum likelihood estimate than the EM algorithm. The latter algorithm converges to the NPMLE if it exists and is unique. The estimation method has been implemented in SAS PROC TCLIFETES or R package `interval`.

To compare survival functions for interval-censored data, one can use a score test based on a regression model for interval-censored data. Several regression models for interval-censored data have been proposed: the grouped proportional hazards model (Finkelstein (1986)), the discrete logistic model (Sun (1996)), and the proportional odds model (Fay (1996)). The survival functions are then compared by performing the score test for $\boldsymbol{\beta} = 0$, where $\boldsymbol{\beta}$ is the vector of regression coefficients for $\boldsymbol{x}_i$. Let $S(t|\boldsymbol{x})$ be the survival function given the covariates $\boldsymbol{x}$. The likelihood function can be written as

$$L(\boldsymbol{\beta}, S_0) = \prod_{i=1}^{n} \sum_{j=1}^{m+1} u_{ij}[S(s_{j-1}|\boldsymbol{x}_i) - S(s_j|\boldsymbol{x}_i)], \tag{4.85}$$

where $u_{ij} = I(s_j \in (L_i, R_i])$. The score test statistic for testing $H_0 : \boldsymbol{\beta} = 0$ is

$$U = \frac{\partial \log L(\boldsymbol{\beta}, \hat{S}_0)}{\partial \boldsymbol{\beta}} \big|_{\boldsymbol{\beta}=0}. \tag{4.86}$$

The score test statistic for each model can be expressed in the same form as the weighted log-rank statistic for right-censored data. Fay and Shaw (2010) showed by simulation that tests by Finkelstein (1986) and Sun (1996) are similar, giving constant weights to differences in survival distribution over time, whereas the test of Fay (1996) gives more weight to early differences. The test of Sun (1996) is closest to the log-rank test for right-censored data, but it does not reduce to the log-rank test for right-censored data. One important drawback of these score-function-based tests is that it is hard to justify the assumptions needed for the regularity conditions for a valid maximum likelihood function. Zhao and Sun (2004) generalized the log-rank test (Sun (1996)) for interval-censored data to include exact failure times. They also used an imputation approach to compute the variance of this generalized log-rank statistic. So et al. (2010) described the use of SAS procedures for analyzing interval-censored survival data. Fay and Shaw (2010) implemented the estimation of survival and weighted log-rank tests for interval censored data.

4.7.1.2   Regression Models for ADA Onset Times

The Cox proportional hazards model (Cox (1972)) is the most commonly used regression model for event-time data with right-censoring. Many have attempted to fit a proportional hazards model to interval-censored data.

Finkelstein (1986) used a discrete survival model, and the estimation is based on a full likelihood under the proportional hazards assumption. The number of parameters might increase with the number of event times, rendering numerically unstable optimization. Goggins et al. (1998) proposed a Monte Carlo EM algorithm to fit the proportional hazard model. Goetghebeur and Ryan (2000) used a different approach which uses an EM algorithm. If the interval-censored time for each subject is a member of a collection of nonoverlapping intervals, the interval-censored data become grouped failure-time data. A multinomial distribution can be used on the number of subjects in the given intervals (Chen et al. (2012)). Prentice and Gloeckler (1978) derived the likelihood for the grouped-data proportional hazards model. The proportional hazards regression for interval-censored data has been implemented in R packages `intcox` (Henschel et al. (2009)) and `ICsurv` (McMahan and Wang (2014)).

4.7.2   Statistical Issues for ADA Duration

4.7.2.1   Persistent and Transient ADA

In addition to the existence of ADA response, one important measure of the ADA response kinetics is the persistence of ADA. It is essentially a dichotomization of the ADA duration. It has been shown that persistent ADA response can be a causal factor of safety issue and may lead to loss of efficacy (Subramanyam (2008)). If an ADA response is drug-induced, but never boosts and eventually disappears due to natural clearance mechanisms, the ADA response is considered as transient. However, there is no consensus on the definition of persistence yet.

Because natural (endogenous) human IgG1, IgG2, and IgG4 have approximate half-lives in the range of 21-25 days, five half-lives are approximately equal to 16 weeks. Shankar et al. (2014) used the following criteria to define the transient and persistent ADA response

- Transient ADA response: Treatment-induced ADA detected only at one time point during the treatment or follow-up period, excluding the last time point, which are considered persistent unless is undetectable in the future or the case detected at two or more time points during the treatment including follow-up period, where gap time between the first and last ADA+ observations is less than 16 weeks, and the subject was ADA− at the last time point.

- Persistent ADA response: Treatment-induced ADA detected at two or more sampling time points during the treatment or follow-up period, where the first and last ADA+ observations are separated by a period of 16 weeks or longer or treatment-induced ADA case only in the last time point or at a time point with less than 16 weeks before the last ADA− observation.

A recent concept paper by the EMA (2014) discussed the strategy of sampling to identify persistent and transient ADA responses. The guideline recommends that for long-term studies, quarterly sampling ensures monitoring for a transient versus a persistent response and maturation to a neutralizing response.

The frequency of sampling and the timing and extent of analyses should depend on the potential risk of a particular drug and the clinical consequences. Sampling schedules should include repeated sampling and be able to distinguish patients with transient or persistent ADA responses. In particular, persistent ADA responses are more critical, since patients with persistent ADA responses are more likely to have clinical consequences in terms of safety and efficacy, while a transient ADA response probably resolves insignificant impact. For biological products intended for chronic use, it is required to assess the evolution and persistence of the ADA responses.

4.7.2.2 Statistical Analysis for Doubly Interval-Censored Data

As a qualitative measurement of ADA duration, classifying ADA responses into persistent versus transient responses results in loss of information. It is more informative to use statistical model to directly characterize the distribution of the duration of ADA responses. Duration of ADA response T is defined as the elapsed time between ADA onset time O and the last ADA+ event time E, i.e., $T = E − O$. Because both onset time and last ADA time can be right- or interval-censored, the ADA duration time is then called doubly-censored (Sun (1998)). Doubly-censored survival data often occurs in epidemiologic studies for disease progression and periodic disease screening. A very popular example arises from the longitudinal study of patients who are at high risk of HIV infection and consequently the development of AIDS. The AIDS incubation time, which is the gap between the HIV infection and the diagnosis of AIDS, is important in the study of progression and prediction of AIDS. For the analysis of doubly-censored survival data with application in HIV studies, see De Gruttola and Lagakos (1989), Bacchetti (1990), Frydman (1992, 1995), Gomez and Lagakos (1994), Jewell (1994), and Jewell et al. (1994).

Because ADA status is identified through periodic immunogenicity tests, the ADA onset times are often interval-censored between the dates of the last

ADA negative test and the first ADA+ test. The last ADA+ time E can be either interval-censored between two consecutive visits or right-censored at the end of study. Therefore, the ADA duration is doubly interval-censored. Here, we briefly discuss the non-parametric estimation of the survival function for doubly censored data. For more discussions about the statistical analysis of doubly interval-censored failure time data, see Sun (1995a,b, 1996); Sun et al. (1999) among others.

Suppose that there are n independent subjects in the study. For the ith subject, let O_i and E_i denote the time of ADA onset and the time of last ADA+ occurrence, respectively. The ADA duration is calculated as $T_i = E_i - O_i$, which is the gap between ADA onset time and the last ADA+ time. Because of the periodic observation scheme of ADA testing, the actual onset and last ADA+ times are not exactly observed. Instead, the ADA event times O_i and E_i are right- or interval-censored. i.e., $O_i \in (L_i, R_i]$ and $E_i \in (U_i, V_i], i = 1, ..., n$. If $L_i = R_i$, then the onset time O_i is exactly observed and the duration time T_i is interval-censored Sun (1998). If $U_i = V_i$ or $V_i = \infty$, the duration time T_i is right-censored. Let $a_1 < \cdots < a_r$ be the mass points for the ADA onset times O_i's and $\tau_1 < \cdots < \tau_s$ be the mass points for the ADA duration. Let $w_j = P(X = a_j), j = 1, ..., r$, and $f_k = P(T = \tau_k), k = 1, ..., s$ be the probability density functions for O and T, respectively. The full likelihood function De Gruttola and Lagakos (1989) for the observed survival data $\{(L_i, R_i], (U_i, V_i], i = 1, ..., n\}$ can be written as:

$$L(w_1, ..., w_r, f_1, ..., f_s) = \prod_{i=1}^{n} \sum_{j=1}^{r} \sum_{k=1}^{s} I(L_i < a_j \leq R_i, U_i < a_j + \tau_k \leq V_i) w_j f_k$$

$$(4.87)$$

The nonparametric maximum likelihood estimator (NPMLE) of the distribution function of T can be computed using the self-consistent algorithm (?). Chen and Zhou (2003) extended the self-consistent algorithm to include a constraint on the NPMLE. They also derived the method for calculating CIs and test hypotheses based on the NPMLE via the empirical likelihood ratio. The estimation method for doubly censored survival data has been implemented in R package `dblcens` (Zhou et al. (2003)). Recently, nonparametric comparison methods of survival functions and semiparametric regression models for doubly-censored survival data have been proposed. For details, see Huang and Wellner (1997), Goggins et al. (1999), Pan (2001) and Sun (2001).

4.7.3 Example

In this example, we compare the distributions of ADA onset times from different dose groups. We classified the subject into two groups according to the doses, i.e., $\leq$ 10mg group and $>$ 10mg group. Because of the discrete ADA testing schedules, the ADA statuses were only identified for week 0 (baseline), and every 4 weeks until week 40 and then every 6 weeks until week 52. Therefore, the ADA onset times are interval-censored. The survival functions of ADA onset times by dose group ($\leq$ 10mg and $>$ 10mg) are shown in Figure 4.7. The survival curves of ADA onset times for the two groups are very close to each other. The rank-based test statistic for the interval-censored times was $U = -0.2684$ with p-value= 0.7884. Therefore, drug dose level was not related to ADA onset times.

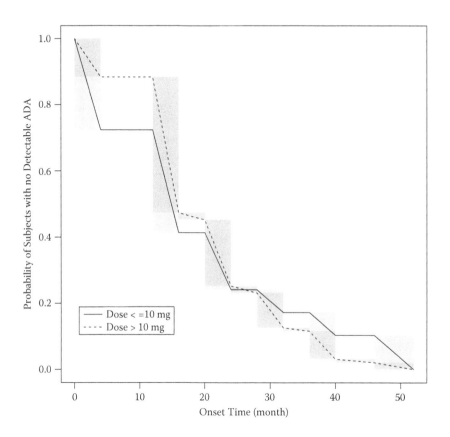

FIGURE 4.7
Survival functions of the ADA onset time by dose group.

4.8 Statistical Analysis of ADA Titer

Although the ADA testing results are often reported as positive versus negative, the ADA magnitude is informative. FDA recommends that positive antibody responses be reported as a titer, which is calculated as the reciprocal of the highest dilution that gives a value equivalent to the cut point of the assay. The titer values may also be reported as amount of drug (in mass units) neutralized per volume serum with the caveat that these are arbitrary *in vitro* assay units and cannot be used to directly assess drug availability *in vivo* (Nauta (2010)).

The ADA titer is usually determined using a titration assay in which a sample containing ADA is serially diluted, e.g., $1/2, 1/4, 1/8, 1/16$ etc. Each dilution is tested for the presence of detectable levels of ADA. The assigned titer value is indicative of the last dilution in which the antibody was detected. For example, if ADA was detected in each of the dilutions listed above, but not in a 1:32 dilution, the titer is said to be 16. If it is detected in the $1 : 2$ and $1 : 4$ dilutions, but no others, the titer is said to be 4. Therefore the titer is a measure of the magnitude of the ADA response.

Assuming that the dilution series is $c_1, c_2, ..., c_K$, then the ADA titers can be categorized in the following three ways (Wang et al. (2002)):

1. When the actual ADA concentration in the sample is so low such that no response is detected at any dilution levels, then the ADA titer is left censored at the lower detection limit (LDL) c_1 and is reported as $< c_1$.

2. When the actual ADA concentration is so high such that antibody responses are detected at all dilution levels, then the ADA titer is right censored at the upper detection limit (UDL) c_K and is often reported as c_k.

3. When the highest dilution level with detectable antibody is achieved among dilution levels $c_1, ..., c_{K-1}$, then the ADA titer is set as $c_k (1 \leq k < K - 1)$. Note that the actual antibody titer lies within an interval $(c_k, c_{k+1}]$.

If we use the standard definition, the ADA titer is determined as the reciprocal of the highest dilution at which the assay response is not detected. The true antibody titer value c actually lies between the standard titer value c_s and the reciprocal of the next dilution c_n, i.e., $c_s \leq c < c_n$. Therefore, the true titer value is underestimated using the standard definition. One approach to correcting the bias is to set antibody titer as $c = \sqrt{c_s c_n}$, if $c_s \leq c < c_n$, which is the middle value of the reciprocals of two serial dilutions (Nauta and de Bruijn (2006); Nauta (2006)).

Like the vaccine clinical trials, the ADA titers are often summarized as geometric means (GMs) (Nauta (2010)). For an ADA titer below the lower detection limit c_1, an imputed value is used in estimating GMs. One commonly used value is half of the detection limit $c_1/2$. Other imputed values include the expected values of order statistics or estimated quantiles. For ADA titers above the lower detection limit c_1, the ADA titers are often set at the middle point. Let $u_1, ..., u_n$ be the ADA titer for the n subjects. The geometric mean titer is defined as

$$GMT = (u_1 \times \cdots \times u_n)^{\frac{1}{n}}. \quad (4.88)$$

The variation of the geometric mean titer is measured by the geometric standard deviation (GSD), which is defined as $GSD = \exp(SD)$, where SD is the standard deviation of the natural logarithm of the ADA titers. Let $\bar{\mu} = \sum_{i=1}^{n} \log(u_i)/n$ and $\widehat{SD} = \sqrt{\sum_{i=1}^{n}(\log u_i - \bar{\mu})^2/(n-1)}$ be the estimates of mean and standard deviation of the log-transformed ADA titers. The two-sided $1 - \alpha$ confidence limits of the mean log-transformed titer μ is

$$(\mu_L, \mu_U) = (\bar{\mu} - t_{1-\alpha/2;n-1}\widehat{SD}/\sqrt{n}, \bar{\mu} + t_{1-\alpha/2;n-1}\widehat{SD}/\sqrt{n}). \quad (4.89)$$

The corresponding confidence limits for the geometric mean $\exp(\bar{\mu})$ can be constructed as $(\exp(\mu_L), \exp(\mu_U))$.

4.8.1 Traditional Analysis of ADA Titers

Nauta (2010) discussed some traditional analysis methods for ADA titers in vaccine trials. The traditional analyses treat the censored or coarse titer values as exactly observed values in estimating GMs. Because the titer values are usually highly skewed, the parametric t-test, which relies on normality assumption for the responses, may not be appropriate. One can use log-transformation to improve symmetry of the distribution of response values. Here, we describe two rank-based statistical methods for comparing the ADA titers between two groups.

The Mann–Whitney (MW) U-test has been applied to two group comparison of ADA titers (Horne (1995)). This test is often used when the responses are not normally distributed, if the variances for the two groups are markedly different or if the responses are on an ordinal scale. The Mann–Whitney U-test ranks the responses from each group and then assesses the difference of rank totals from the two groups.

Let $d_{1i}, i = 1, ..., n_1$ be the ADA titers for Group 1 and $d_{2i}, i = 1, ..., n_2$ be the ADA titers for Group 2. Let the distribution functions for the titer values from the two groups denoted by F_1 and F_2, respectively. Assume that the distribution F_1 is a shift relative the distribution F_2, i.e., $F_1(u) = F_2(u + \theta)$. The Mann–Whitney U-test can be used to test the null hypothesis $H_0 : F_1 = F_2$ versus $H_0 : F_1 \neq F_2$. The U-statistic is calculated as

$$U = \sum_{i=1}^{n_1} \sum_{j=1}^{n_2} \left[I(d_{2j} > d_{1i}) + \frac{1}{2}I(d_{1i} = d_{2j}) \right]. \quad (4.90)$$

The null hypothesis of equal distribution will be rejected if U is too large or too small. The Wilcoxon rank-sum statistic differs from the MW U-statistics by a constant factor (Hollander and Wolfe (1999)). For this reason, the test is sometimes called Wilcoxon–Mann–Whitney (WMW) test.

For comparison of ADA titers among multiple independent groups, one can use Kruskal–Wallis (KW) test (Hollander and Wolfe (1999)). The KW test is most commonly used to test the association between a nominal categorical variable and a continuous response variable, and the distribution of the response variable does not necessarily meet the normality assumption. It is the nonparametric analogue of the one-way ANOVA. A one-way ANOVA model may yield inaccurate estimates of the p-value when the data are not normally distributed. The KW test is calculated by combining responses from all G groups and ranking them among all observations in the combined data. Then the total ranks within each group are calculated. Under the null hypothesis $H_0 : F_1 = F_2 = \cdots = F_G$, the rank sums for the G groups are expected to be similar. The Kruskal–Wallis statistic is a weighted sum of squared difference between the observed and expected rank sums:

$$K = \frac{12}{N(N+1)} \sum_{i=1}^{G} \frac{1}{n_i} \left[R_i - \frac{n_i(N+1)}{2} \right]^2, \qquad (4.91)$$

where R_i is the observed rank sum for the ith group, $N = \sum_{i=1}^{G} n_i$ is the total sample size and $n_i(N+1)/2$ is the expected rank sum. When the sample sizes are relatively large for each group, the distribution of K under the null hypothesis can be approximated as a chi-square distribution with $G-1$ degrees of freedom.

4.8.2   Maximum Likelihood Method for ADA Titer

Because of the discrete nature of serial dilution and the limit of detection, the ADA titer values cannot be exactly observed. Treating the ADA titer as exact values may cause bias and underestimate the variance of titers. Therefore, alternative methods have been recommended to model ADA titer (Wang et al. (2002); Moulton and Halsey (1995); Bonate et al. (2009); Zaccaro and Aertker (2011)).

Let Y denote the random variable for the latent (unobserved) titer value, which follows a lognormal (LN) distribution $Y \sim LN(\mu, \sigma^2)$, where μ is the mean and σ is the standard deviation of the log-transformed titer. Let $y_1, ..., y_n$ be the latent titer values for n subjects. Because of the serial dilution assay format, the exact value of y_i's fall into on of the following intervals $\Delta_0 = [0, d_1), \Delta_1 = [d_1, d_2), \cdots, \Delta_{K-1} = [d_{K-1}, d_K), \Delta_K = [d_K, \infty)$. The mean and standard deviation of the titers can be estimated using the maximum likelihood method.

Based on the lognormal assumption for the ADA titer, the probabilities of

Y falling into interval Δ_k's are

$$
\begin{aligned}
P_0 &= P(Y \in [0, d_1)) = \Phi\left(\frac{\log d_1 - \mu}{\sigma}\right) \\
P_k &= P(Y \in [d_k, d_{k+1})) = \Phi\left(\frac{\log d_{k+1} - \mu}{\sigma}\right) - \Phi\left(\frac{\log d_k - \mu}{\sigma}\right), \\
&\quad k = 1, ..., K - 1, \\
P_K &= P(Y \in [d_K, \infty)) = 1 - \Phi\left(\frac{\log d_K - \mu}{\sigma}\right).
\end{aligned}
$$

Let $\mathbf{I}_i = (I_{i1}, ..., I_{i,K})$ be the vector of interval indicators for the ith subject, where $I_{ik} = I(y_i \in \Delta_k), k = 0, ..., K$. The likelihood function for observed data $(\mathbf{I}_1, ..., \mathbf{I}_n)$ is

$$
L(\mu, \sigma) = \prod_{i=1}^{n} \prod_{k=0}^{K} P_k^{I_{ik}} \tag{4.92}
$$

The MLEs of (μ, σ) of interval-censored titer data from a lognormal distribution can be obtained using SAS PROC LIFEREG.

To compare the median titers from two groups or to examine the association between median titer and the covariates, one can assume a linear regression model for the location parameter μ

$$
\mu = \alpha + \beta x, \tag{4.93}
$$

where x is the group indicator or explanatory variables. The difference between the two groups can be measured by β.

4.8.3 Nonparametric Method for Comparing ADA Titers

Wilcoxon-type rank test can also be used to test the difference of interval-censored ADA titers (Fay and Shaw (2010)). The weighted log-rank tests are developed for interval censored survival data and have been described in previous sections for ADA onset times. The statistical methods for interval-censored data can be used for ADA titer analysis. We briefly describe an alternative score test for comparing ADA titers.

Let c_i be the observed titer value for the ith subject. Denote the distribution function for the ADA titer as $F(c_i|x_i, \beta, \gamma) = P(y_i > c_i|x_i)$, where x_i is the covariate for the ith subject, β is the vector of treatment parameters and γ is the vector of nuisance parameters for the unknown distribution function. The ADA titer can be modeled as

$$
\log(y_i) = \alpha + \beta x_i + \sigma \epsilon_i, \tag{4.94}
$$

where α is the intercept and β is the vector of regression coefficients and the random errors follow a known distribution F_0, say normal or logistic. The likelihood function for interval-censored data is

$$L = \prod_{i=1}^{n} \left[F(R_i|x_i, \theta) - F(L_i|x_i, \theta) \right]. \tag{4.95}$$

The score statistic can be derived by taking the derivative of $\log(L)$ with respect to parameter β and evaluate it at $\beta = 0$. The resulting score test has been implemented in R package `interval` with the option scores=`"logranks1"` (Fay and Shaw (2010)).

4.8.4 Longitudinal Modeling of ADA Titer

In clinical trials for biological products, most patients do not have ADA reactions, so the ADA titers are either zero or under the detection limit. A zero-inflated Poisson (ZIP) model has been used for ADA titers with many 0's. In a longitudinal clinical trial, ADA titer values are observed repeatedly over time for each subject. In this situation, a ZIP random-effects model can be used (Bonate et al. (2009)).

The ADA titer is formulated as a geometric sequence $u_{ij} = a \times b^{Y_{ij}}$, where a is the scale factor that is equal to half limit of detection and b is the dilution factor. For example, for a serial dilution assay with a detection limit 10 and dilution factor 2, the ADA titer can be expressed as $10 = 5 \times 2^1, 20 = 5 \times 2^2$ etc. ADA titers that are less than the detection limit of 2 can take the value of $Y_{ij} = 0$. As ADA titer data from clinical trials typically show an excess of zeros. The random-effects ZIP model can be formulated as:

$$P(Y_{ij} = m | \boldsymbol{x}_{ij}, \boldsymbol{z}_{ij}, \boldsymbol{b}_i) = \begin{cases} \pi_{ij} + (1 - \pi_{ij}) \exp(-\lambda_{ij}) & m = 0 \\ (1 - \pi_{ij}) \frac{\exp(-\lambda_{ij})\lambda_{ij}^m}{m!} & m > 0 \end{cases}, \tag{4.96}$$

where π_{ij} is the excess probability of being zero and λ_{ij} is the mean of the Poisson count. The parameters (π_{ij}, λ_{ij}) can be modeled as

$$\log \left(\frac{\pi_{ij}}{1 - \pi_{ij}} \right) = \beta_\pi \boldsymbol{x}_{ij} + \boldsymbol{b}_{\pi i} \boldsymbol{z}_{ij}$$
$$\lambda_{ij} = \exp(\beta_\lambda \boldsymbol{x}_{ij} + \boldsymbol{b}_{\lambda i} \boldsymbol{z}_{ij}).$$

where $\boldsymbol{x}_{ij}$ is the vector of covariates for the fixed effects β_λ and β_π and $\boldsymbol{z}_{ij}$ is the vector of covariates for the random effects $\boldsymbol{b}_{\pi i}$ and $\boldsymbol{b}_{\lambda i}$. The random-effects ZIP model can be fitted using SAS PROC NLMIXED.

4.8.5 Example

In this example, we continued to examine the magnitude of ADA titer and the impact of dose level on ADA titer for the 135 subjects who are ADA positive. The mean and median unadjusted ADA titer of the four groups are shown in Table 4.16. The mean titers are much higher than the median titers. This

TABLE 4.16

Unadjusted mean and median ADA titer by dose group

Group	n	Mean ADA titer	Median ADA titer
Placebo	8	258	120
10 mg	25	369	80
20 mg	40	473	160
40 mg	60	493	160

is because the titer values are typically extremely right skewed. Therefore, a log-transformation was applied to the original titer values. The histogram of the log-transformed ADA titers is shown in Figure 4.8.

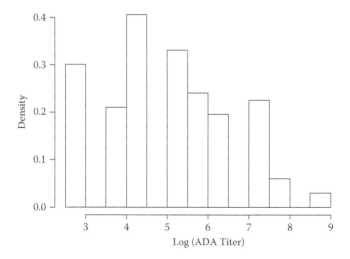

FIGURE 4.8

Histogram of the logarithm of ADA titer.

In Table 4.16, we also notice that the mean titers increased with dose levels. The rank-based score statistic for interval-censored data was 37.8 with p-value < 0.001. The ADA titers were significantly associated with dose level. As described in Section 4.8.2, the estimated mean and median titers based on the raw titer values are biased. We also used a maximum likelihood method

TABLE 4.17
Estimates of ADA titers by dose group from the likelihood method

| Group | n | Mean ADA titer | | Median ADA titer | |
		Mean	95% CI	Median	95% CI
Placebo	8	370	137 999	135	50 364
10 mg	25	484	276 850	176	100 310
20 mg	40	690	442 1076	251	161 392
40 mg	60	674	469 969	245	171 353

to estimate the median titer values. Specifically, we assume a lognormal distribution for the titer values. The observed titer value is $[L_i, R_i)$ for the ith subject with dose level x_i and the lognormal model for the titer assumes that $y_i \in [L_i, R_i)$ and

$$\log(y_i) = \alpha + \beta x_i + \sigma \epsilon_i, \epsilon_i \sim N(0, 1) \qquad (4.97)$$

The estimates of mean and median ADA titers from the lognormal model were shown in Table 4.17. The estimates of mean and median ADA titers based on the likelihood method were different from the crude estimates based on the raw titer values.

4.9 Meta-Analysis

Meta-analysis is a quantitative synthesis method that combines results from multiple studies (Glass (1976)). In clinical trials, meta-analysis is often used to assess the efficacy and safety of a new treatment or drug (Stangl and Berry (2000); Whitehead (2002)). A meta-analysis aggregates and contrasts findings from multiple related studies, often with a systematic literature review. For example, individual small clinical trials may fail to show a statistically significant difference between the treatment and control groups because of small sample size or inefficient study design. By pooling the results from the multiple studies using appropriate synthesis method, one can demonstrate the treatment effect with higher power (DerSimonian and Laird (1986); DerSimonian and Kacker (2007)). Depending on the nature and the endpoint of studies, a wide range of techniques can be used for meta-analysis, including the attributable risk, hazard ratio and relative risk (Fleiss and Berlin (2009)).

By combining results from many moderate or even small trials, meta-analysis have more power to detect small but clinically significant treatment effect. In addition, meta-analysis can be used to detect the heterogeneity of the treatment effects among different studies. There are still many pitfalls in performing a valid meta-analysis. An unsystematic review, which only includes a portion of relevant studies by accident or excludes critical studies with inappropriate inclusion criteria, may introduce systematic inclusion bias (Walker et al. (2008)). Another concern is the publication bias, as clinical trials that show no beneficial treatment effect or negative scientific findings are less likely to get published (Thornton and Lee (2000)). Therefore, a comphrensive meta-analyses should have complete coverage of all relevant studies, look for the presence of heterogeneity, and explore the robustness of the main findings using sensitivity analysis. Recently, meta-analysis has been extended to examine the AEs (Lievre et al. (2002); Vandermeer et al. (2009)). For extensive discussions and applications of meta-analysis, see Whitehead (2002) and Chen and Peace (2013).

4.9.1 Fixed-Effects and Random-Effects Models

When using fixed-effects models, the goal is to make a conditional inference based on the multiple studies included in the analysis (Hedges and Vevea (1998)). Often a weighted least-squares model is used. The estimate of overall effect from the weighted least-squares model is calculated as

$$\bar{\theta}_w = \frac{\sum_i w_i \theta_i}{\sum_i w_i} \qquad (4.98)$$

where w_i's are the weights of the studies. On the other hand, unweighted least-squares provides an estimate of

$$\bar{\theta} = \frac{\sum_i \theta_i}{K}. \qquad (4.99)$$

the simple unweighted average of the true effects.

The random-effects model for the meta-analysis assumes that the observed study effects come from a random distribution for the effect population (DerSimonian and Laird (1986); DerSimonian and Kacker (2007)). Let $y_1, ..., y_k$ be the estimates of effect size from K independent studies. The random-effects model assumes that

$$y_i = \theta_i + e_i, i = 1, ...k, \qquad (4.100)$$

where y_i denotes the observed effect in the ith study, θ_i the unknown true effect, $e_i \sim N(0; v_i)$ is the error term. The observed effects y_i's are unbiased and normally distributed. The sampling variances v_i's are assumed to be known. Depending on the outcome measure used, a bias correction, normalizing, and/or variance stabilizing transformation may be necessary to ensure that these assumptions are approximately true. For example, a log transformation can be used for odds ratios and Fisher's z transformation can be used for correlations.

Differences in the methods and sample characteristics may introduce variability among the true treatment effects. One way to model the heterogeneity is to treat θ_i's as random effects.

$$\theta_i = \mu + u_i \qquad (4.101)$$

where $u_i \sim N(0; \tau_2)$. Therefore, the true effects are assumed to be normally distributed with mean 0 and variance τ^2. The goal is then to estimate μ, the average true effect and τ^2 the total amount of heterogeneity among the true effects.

In contrast to the fixed-effects model, the random-effects models provide an unconditional inference about a larger set of studies from which the multiple studies included are assumed to be a random sample from the population (Hedges and Vevea (1998)). The hypothetical population of studies comprises studies that have been conducted, that could have been conducted, or that may be conducted in the future. Jackson et al. (2010) compared the efficiency of the random-effects model and other related methods for meta-analysis. The random-effects model for meta-analysis can be estimated using SAS PROC MIXED or R function *lmer*. In addition, quite a few R packages, e.g., `meta` and `metafor` (Viechtbauer (2010)), are available for standard meta-analysis.

Meta-analysis can also be used to summarize the incidence, prevalence of ADA responses and to estimate the effects of ADA response on efficacy and safety. For example, Maneiro et al. (2013) summarized the influence of ADA response against biologic agents on efficacy and safety in immune-mediated inflammatory diseases. Garcês et al. (2013) assessed the effect of ADA on drug response to infliximab, adalimumab, and etanercept, and the effect of immunosuppression on ADA detection, in patients with RA, Spondyloarthritis, Psoriasis and Inflammatory Bowel Diseases.

4.9.2 Example

ADA response of anti-TNF drugs is one of the mechanisms behind treatment failure. Garcês et al. (2013) showed that detectable ADA reaction reduced the drug response rate. Using the data for the effect of ADA on drug response for the RA patients, we fit a random-effects model to estimate the relative risk of the drug response rates by ADA status from different studies. The forest plot including the relative risk for the studies for RA is shown in Figure 4.9. The results show that the estimate of average log-relative risk is -0.56 with 95% CI $(-0.80, -0.33)$. This indicates that the patients with detectable ADA have significantly lower response rates. Therefore, the meta-analysis shows that having ADA significantly reduces the drug efficacy.

Several measures were used to estimate the heterogeneity among the studies. The I^2 statistic is an estimate of the total variability in the effect size estimates, which consists of both heterogeneity and sampling variability. When $I^2 = 0\%$ or $\hat{\tau}^2 = 0$, the study results are perfectly homogeneous. The H^2 statistic is the ratio of the total amount of variability in the observed outcomes to the amount of sampling variability. The estimates of τ^2 was $\hat{\tau}^2 = 0.0322$ with standard error 0.0565, and the estimates for I^2 and H^2 were 31.70% and 1.46, respectively. The Q-test used to test heterogeneity has test statistic 12.345 with p-value 0.09, indicating a borderline significant heterogeneity among the RR's from different studies.

Author, year	ADA+		ADA–			RR (95% CI)
	R	N	R	N		
Bender 2007	4	13	2	2		−0.95 [−1.87, −0.04]
Radstake 2009	0	10	24	24		−3.07 [−5.78, −0.36]
Bartelds 2011	47	76	168	196		−0.33 [−0.51, −0.14]
Pascual–Salcedo 2011	9	16	29	33		−0.45 [−0.90, 0.00]
Radstake 2009	4	18	17	17		−1.41 [−2.22, −0.60]
Pascual–Salcedo 2011	4	7	23	24		−0.52 [−1.16, 0.13]
Wolbink 2006	8	22	20	29		−0.64 [−1.24, −0.04]
Pascual–Salcedo 2011	6	11	33	36		−0.52 [−1.07, 0.03]
RE Model						−0.56 [−0.80, −0.33]

```
                    −6.00      −2.00      2.00
                       Log Relative Risk
```

FIGURE 4.9

Forest plot of the relative risk of ADA on responder rates.

5

Immunogenicity Risk Control

CONTENTS

5.1 Introduction

Risk management is a systematic process of identifying, assessing and controlling risks, and communicating the outcomes to all stakeholders in a timely manner. Risk management principles have been effectively utilized in many areas of business and government to facilitate decision-making in the face of risks and uncertainty. Although utilization of such strategies is commonplace in finance, insurance, occupational safety, public health, pharmacovigilance, and by agencies regulating these industries, it was not until the publication of several ICH documents (ICH Q8, ICH Q9, and ICH Q10) at the turn of 2000 did the pharmaceutical industry start adopting the method. Successful utilization of risk management principles has led to development of highly efficacious biopharmaceuticals and robust manufacturing processes (Rathore and Mhatre (2011)). As outlined in ICH Q9, risk management has several key components, including risk assessment, control, and communication. A typical risk management process is shown in Figure 5.1.

All therapeutic proteins have the potential to be immunogenic. In recent years, a risk-based approach to immunogenicity risk assessment has been proposed by researchers in both industry and regulatory agencies (Koren et al. (2008), FDA (2013), EMA (2007, 2012, 2013)). The essential components of a risk-based approach to immunogenicity assessment encompass determining (1) the molecular characteristics of the therapeutic protein; (2) the mechanism of action (MOA) and intended use of the protein; (3) target population; (4) risk factors including those factors discussed in Chapter 1; (5) associated risk control strategies (Koren et al. (2008)). The knowledge of the protein's molecular characteristics, MOA, therapeutic indication, and intended recipients helps classify the molecule into lower, moderate, or high risk category. Such classification forms the basis for the development of ADA testing plan including sampling time and frequency during clinical development. For example, the more immunogenic the molecule is, the more frequent the ADA testing needs to be conducted. Identifying and assessing the criticality of risk factors is an integral part of overall immunogenicity risk management. For this purpose, prior knowledge of laboratory, nonclinical data, and clinical experience can be utilized. Once the risk factors are identified and risk level determined, proper control strategies can be devised.

It is also well recognized that the risk varies considerably from product to product. As a result, it is possible that a factor that has the potential to increase immunogenic risk in one product may not be a risk factor for other products. Since immunogenicity is a very complex phenomenon, it needs to be dealt with from a holistic perspective applying the full risk-based approach recommended in regulatory guidelines on each and every product. Suffice to say, approaching immunogenicity risk based on risk management methodologies and principles is essential in the effective mitigation of such risk.

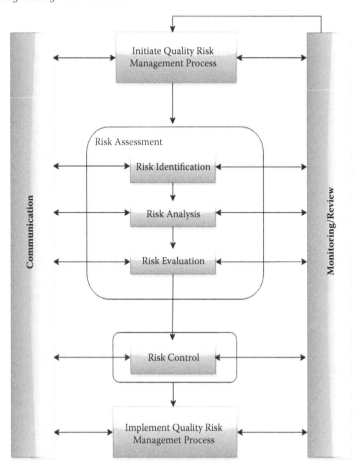

FIGURE 5.1

Process of quality risk management.

The first step toward risk control is to identify all immunogenic risk factors, analyze, and determine their criticality, which is defined as impact on clinical safety and efficacy. The criticality determination is the basis for developing and implementing appropriate risk control strategies. Risk management is an evolving and dynamic process, and relies on information collected during the life cycle of the product under development. As new knowledge of immunogenicity of the product is being obtained during product development, it should be incorporated into the original risk management decision. Therefore, the output/result of the quality risk management process should be communicated and reviewed on an ongoing basis to account for new knowledge. In general the method should be consistent with risk management principles and methodologies outlined in ICH Q9. Many tools listed in the guidance such as failure model effects analysis (FMEA), risk ranking and filtering, statistical methods including control charts and design of experiment (DOE) can be used to support and facilitate development of a risk-based approach to immunogenicity risk assessment.

This chapter focuses on statistical methods that can be utilized to conduct comprehensive risk assessment and develop control strategies. Simple but useful tools such as fishbone diagram and Pareto plot are introduced to facilitate initial identification of risk factors. More sophisticated statistical methods including various modeling and data dimension reduction techniques are also discussed. They have the potential to provide greater control over immunogenicity risk. Although it might be challenging to implement these multivariate methods, proper statistical algorithms can be developed and validated to make them accessible to lay users. Some implementations are discussed in relative detail in Chapter 6.

5.2 Risk Assessment

5.2.1 Identification of Risk Factors

The cumulative experience with biopharmaceutical development has generated a huge body of knowledge concerning immunogenicity risk factors (Rosenberg and Worobec (2004a,b, 2005)). For a therapeutic protein under development, critical examination of the available data is an important step in culling risk factors. Relevant scientific considerations need to be given when assessing risk factors. For example, if the therapeutic has a non-redundant endogenous counterpart, it should be listed as a risk factor. As pointed out by many researchers (van de Weert and Møller (2008)), aggregation is of primary concern as an immunogenicity risk factor. However, its actual impact depends on structure of the product. Whether they are immune-stimulatory or immune-modulatory also has impact on their immunogenic potential. Such knowledge needs to be taken into account in identification of risk factors. In addition, published regulatory guidance (EMA (2007), FDA (2013)) also provide helpful insights on potential risk factors that should be considered in immunogenicity risk assessment. Identification of potential immunogenicity risk factors pertinent to a specific drug may start with addressing a set of well-structured questions such as those by Chamberlain (2008, 2011).

As previously discussed, risk factors can be product-related, process-related, patient-related characteristics, and treatment-related factors, which sometimes are referred to as product-extrinsic factors. However, the case-specific nature of immunogenicity risk makes it necessary to map out and organize potential risk factors in a manner that facilitates risk assessment. For this purpose, a fishbone or Ishikawa diagram (Ishikawa (1982)) can be used for dissecting cause and effect, depicting all the potential risk factors of immunogenicity. Such diagrams created and popularized by Ishikawa in late

1960s is a useful risk management tool displaying causes of a specific effect of interest. It allows one to cull factors causing an overall effect. On the diagram, causes are grouped into various categories, representing different sources of impact on the total effect. Figure 5.2 displays a fishbone diagram, showing the relationships between the potential risk factors on immunogenicity risk. Factors are grouped in product-related, process-related, patient-related, and treatment-related categories. In practice, factors within each group can be further grouped into smaller categories, to add more granularities in the cause effect analysis.

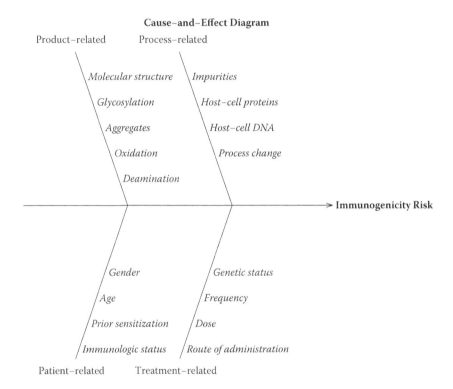

FIGURE 5.2
An example of a fishbone diagram.

5.2.2 Criticality of Risk Factors

Following the initial culling of risk factors, a formal risk assessment is carried out for each potential risk factor such as aggregation and impurity with the intent to determine its criticality. In ICH Q9 "Quality Risk Management", it is stated "It is commonly understood that risk is defined as the combination of the probability of occurrence of harm and the severity of that harm." As a result, the first step in a risk factor criticality assessment is to determine both severity of immunogenicity due to the risk factor and probability or likelihood for the immunogenic event to occur. The severity ranks the risk factor based on the consequences of immunogenic reaction; whereas likelihood characterizes the probability for an immunogenic event to occur when the risk factor is outside of its acceptable range. Severity ranking is typically discrete. It is intimately related to both the impact and uncertainty of the potential risk factor on immunogenicity. A high impact is considered highly severe, so is an unknown risk. Appropriate expertise and other prior knowledge are essential in assigning impact and uncertainty scores. The severity score can be calculated as the product of impact score and uncertainty score. In recent years, this risk ranking method has been used in bioprocess development. Two noted examples are case studies by two working groups (CMC Biotech Working Group (2009), CMC Vaccine Working Group (2012)). The risk ranking method is essential for the identification of risk factors, which impact product immunogenicity. An example of severity score calculation is given in Table 5.1 (CMC Biotech Working Group (2009)). The impact score has three levels, 2, 8, and 25 while the uncertainty has 5 levels, 1-5. Potential severity scores are listed. Determination of both impact and uncertainty scores is driven by scientific knowledge of the product and process, requiring contributions from personnel in multiple disciplines.

TABLE 5.1

Determination of severity scores

Impact	Uncertainty				
	1	2	3	4	5
2	2	4	6	8	10
8	8	16	24	32	40
25	25	50	75	100	125

Alternatively, one may directly assign severity score to one of a few numerical values, based on a mutually agreed upon severity definition such as that listed in Table 5.2.

However, the probability of occurrence can be either discrete or continuous, and can often be determined through analyzing pre-clinical and clinical data. Methods discussed in Chapter 4 make it possible to estimate probability of immunogenicity occurrence due to a particular risk factor, assuming adequate data are available. This might require one to synthesize information from various data sources, based on meta-analysis. Probabilities derived from statistical models are usually continuous. In the absence of data from well-designed studies, expert knowledge can be used to assign probabilities values.

Table 5.3 provides an example from the A-MAb study (CMC Biotech Working Group (2009)).

TABLE 5.2
Severity definition

Severity Score	Severity Definition
11–125	Very high– death, hypersensitive immune reaction
8–10	High – serious immunogenic response
6	Moderate – moderate immunogenicity or reduction in efficacy
4	Low – low immunogenicity or small reduction in
2	Very low – no measurable impact

TABLE 5.3
Likelihood definition

Likelihood Score	Likelihood of Severity
9	Very high
7	High
5	Moderate
3	Low
1	Very low

After the severity ranking and probability of an immunogenic event are elicited, a risk score is calculated as the product of severity and likelihood. When the risk of all factors is quantified, factors that have greater potential to cause immunogenicity are determined based on a cutoff of the risk score. A factor is considered critical if its risk score is above this cutoff value. Selection of the cutoff is critical as a too low value would result in too many non-critical factors being classified as critical and a too high value would run the risk of misclassifying critical factors. There are several methods that can be considered to aid determination of the cutoff. The first is to rank the risk scores from smallest to the highest, and set the cutoff to be equal to the smallest risk score among the scores of those which are deemed critical, based on prior knowledge. Another method is to use a Pareto plot. Risk scores are plotted, along with the curve of the cumulative total effect and cutoff line of 80% for the cumulative total effect. Factors of larger risk scores that make up the 80% of the total contribution are considered to be critical. The plot is based on the Pareto principle which states that among all the causes that may have effects on an outcome, roughly 20% of them cause 80% of the effects (Bunkley (2008)). Take as an example, suppose we have the risk scores for the factors, immunologic status, prior sensitization, route of administration, genetic status, endogenous protein, product origin, post translational modification, aggregates, glycosylation, impurity, immunomodulatory properties, formulation, container closure, and product custody, which are 2, 4, 6, 8, 125, 8, 25, 50, 75, 100, 40, 24, 24, and 16, respectively. A Pareto plot is constructed and shown in Figure 5.3. Risk scores of the 14 factors are displayed from the largest to the smallest. The curve represents the percent of cumulative total risk score while the horizontal line is the value of 80% of the total risk score. From the plot, it is evident that risk factors of endogenous protein, impurity, glycosylation, aggregates, and immunomodulatory properties account for about 80% of the total risk scores. Therefore, they are potential risk factors, when compared to the others.

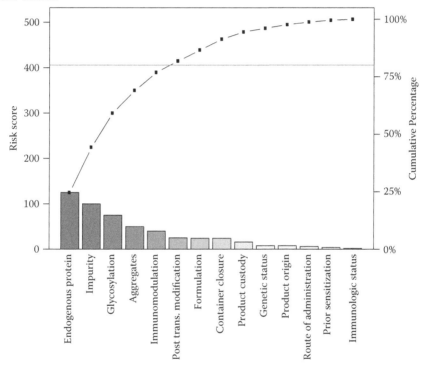

FIGURE 5.3

Pareto plot of potential risk factors. The curve is the cumulative risk score and the horizontal line is the risk score of 80% of the total risk score.

The result of the above criticality analysis is used to guide the development of suitable test plan and appropriate control of the factors. It is conceivable that the more knowledge of the potential risk factors is gained from *in vitro*, *in silico*, and *in vivo* studies including both animal and human trials, the easier it is to develop a risk mitigation plan. It is also worth pointing out that factors which are deemed to be less critical because their risk scores are below the cutoff should be carefully reviewed to evaluate if their categorizations are consistent with other products in the same class. For example, host cell DNA may be judged to be a less critical risk factor, using the data pertinent to the therapeutic protein. However, if host cell DNA has been shown to be immunogenic for proteins in the same class, the information may be used to calibrate the criticality assessment of host cell DNA for the current protein.

5.3 Immunogenicity Risk Control

After the risk factors are identified and their criticality determined, a risk management plan should be developed. It is important to bear in mind that immunogenicity risk control is multifactorial, involving many considerations. It may involve a testing plan that mitigates risk through ADA monitoring, methods and technique that make the molecule less immunogenic, control of multiple product and process-related risk factors to reduce product immuno-genic responses, and selection of sub-population of patients that are less prone to adverse immune responses.

To devise proper clinical sample testing plan, it is necessary to determine the overall risk. The overall risk, possibly having the classification of low, medium, or high risk, serves as a rationale for ADA testing scheme, in terms of sampling timing and frequency, extent of ADA characterizations. An ADA risk management plan is provided by Koren et al. (2008). For low risk molecules, the plan only requires screening for ADAs at baseline and end of study, and testing for drug-specific IgE if only hypersensitivity reactions are suspected or observed. However, for molecules deemed to be of moderate risk, screening for ADAs at baseline, Day 14, monthly, and bi-monthly is recommended in addition to testing for neutralizing ADA should efficacy be reduced. Lastly for high risk molecules, the screening for ADA should be carried out with higher regularity and after drug washout. It is also necessary to test screening positive samples for both IgG and IgM, and neutralizing ADAs. As pointed out by Koren et al. (2008), the greater the immunogenicity of the molecule, the more necessary it is to conduct extensive and frequent ADA testing and characterization, along with other clinical pre-cautions.

A broad range of techniques have been developed to reduce immunogenic-ity risk, including modification of the therapeutic protein structure, human-izing the therapeutic protein, clinical measures, etc. Covalent attachment of polyethylene glycol (PEG) to the therapeutic molecule has been shown to be effective in extending the molecule's half-life, reducing the chance of immune response (van de Weert and Møller (2008)). Immunosuppression through treat-ment inhibiting T-cell responses, induction of immune tolerance to therapeu-tic protein using large doses, and removal of T-cell epitope of the therapeutic molecule all have the potential to counter unwanted immune responses.

For product and process-related risk factors, immunogenicity risk can be reduced by ensuring that the risk factors are controlled within acceptable ranges. Establishment of such ranges relies on data collected during the life cycle of the product, including those from preclinical and clinical trials, stability studies, and process validation, and often requires application of appropriate statistical methods. It is also essential to link the ranges to immunogenicity risk through probability of occurrence and severity. By mitigating probability of immunogenicity and/or severity, the risk attributable to a particular CMC factors can be controlled to an acceptable level.

Immunogenicity is a complex phenomenon. Apart from the consensus that ADA formation is the marker for immunogenicity, there has been little effort in identifying markers that can help segment patients into groups that are more or less prone to produce immune responses against therapeutic proteins. This is potentially caused by the facts (1) that data from pre-clinical studies have limited utility in predicting immune responses; (2) clinical experience and data are limited when a product is under development; and (3) segmentation of patients based on information synthesized from multiple sources can be very challenging. However, statistical modeling, simulation, and inference concern themselves with "learning from data" to "translating data into knowledge" in a disciplined, robust and reproducible way. They have been shown to be a powerful tool for identifying markers for drug safety and efficacy. If properly applied, statistical modeling, simulation, and inference can link patient characteristic to immune responses, and distinguish patients who are more likely to have devastating immune responses from others.

As noted in ICH Q9, new risks may be introduced due to the implementation of risk reduction measures. Hence, risk assessment is not a static process. Instead, it should continue through the lifecycle of a product development. It is necessary to identify and evaluate any possible change in risk after implementing a risk reduction process. It is also worth noting that a successful immunogenicity risk management plan is likely to include a multitude of strategies described above.

In the following, we concentrate on controlling immunogenicity through development of acceptable ranges for key risk factors, and segmentation of the patient population to focus on a subset of the population that has less potential to have adverse immune response to the treatment. Relevant statistical methods are introduced, and illustrated through case examples.

5.3.1   Acceptance Range

The acceptance ranges of risk factors are a region such that movement within the range will not cause unacceptable level of unwanted immunogenicity. In theory, the region can be determined through DOEs in which the relationship between immune responses and risk factors are evaluated. The most relevant data are those collected from clinical studies, including ADA-related adverse events. However, at the time of risk assessment, clinical experience is usually limited. As a result, statistical models such as logistic regression are often used to explore the relationship between immunogenicity events and risk factors of interest. Often, the acceptance ranges of risk factors are established separately, forming a hypercube in a multi-dimensional space. Immunogenicity risk is under control when the risk factors are confined within the hypercube. Figure 5.4 displays such a region for aggregation and impurity. The rectangle area corresponds to drug substance lots satisfying $0 \leq$ drug aggregation $\leq a$, and $0 \leq$ drug impurity $\leq b$.

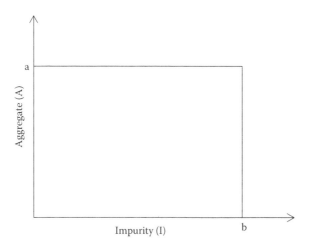

FIGURE 5.4
Acceptance range of drug substance aggregate and impurity when aggregate and impurity do not have any joint effect on product immunogenicity.

One potential pitfall of this method is that the acceptance region is determined for each risk factor in isolation, without taking into account the potential correlation among the factors. For example, for certain products, drug substance impurity and aggregation may produce a joint effect on immunogenicity. In other words, with less aggregation, a product with a high level of impurity may have a more acceptable immunogenicity profile than those with a higher level of aggregate. Because the degree to which drug aggregate impacts the drug immunogenicity depends in part on impurity, understanding the relationship is critical to simultaneously set appropriate acceptance ranges for both attributes. It is also conceivable that the simultaneous control limits for drug aggregate and impurity are likely to take a geometric shape different from a rectangle. Figure 5.5 depicts an acceptable region for drug aggregate and impurity when the two risk factors have a joint effect on immunogenicity. The dependence between the drug aggregate and impurity is characterized by the specification of drug aggregate which has a decreasing linear relationship with the drug impurity. Thus, to offset the effect of increased impurity, less aggregation is necessary to minimize unacceptable level of immune responses compared to the cases where lower level of impurity is present.

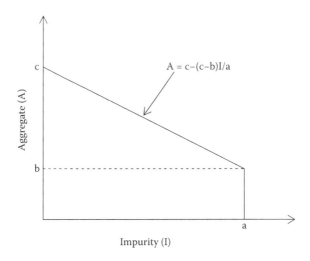

FIGURE 5.5
Specifications of drug substance aggregate and impurity when aggregate and impurity have a joint effect on product immunogenicity.

As noted by several researchers (Yang (2013), Peterson (2008)), the correlation structure of quality attributes can have an important influence on the probability of meeting specification. For example, suppose that the measurements of drug aggregate y_1 and impurity (%) y_2 follows a bivariate normal distribution with mean of $(100, 10)$ and variance of $(20^2, 2^2)$. Let ρ denote the correlation between concentration and impurity. It is also assumed that the specifications of drug concentration and impurity are $(80, 120)$ and $(0, 11)$, respectively. It can be calculated that the probabilities for the both measurements to fall in their respective specifications are 0.5023 and 0.4736 for $\rho = -0.75$ and 0, respectively. The example showed that specifications based on one set of assumptions of correlation structure among the quality attributes may not render the same level of quality assurance when the true correlation structure is different from what is used to set the specifications. Hence, it is important to account for the correlations among quality attributes when establishing specifications. This requires simultaneously linking risk factors to drug immunogenicity when inter-dependence exists among the quality attributes.

5.3.2 Case Example

In this section, through an example we demonstrate how to control immunogenicity risk due to unmethylated CpG motifs in residual host cell DNA, and develop control strategies to minimize such risk. The product is a vaccine manufactured in Madin Darby Canine Kidney (MDCK) cells. To reduce the risk of residual DNA, multiple purification steps are utilized to reduce the content of residual DNA. Two processes, tangential flow filtration (TFF) and chromatography assay, are employed sequentially. The former removes DNA from the virus, based on the size difference between the virus and host cell DNA while the latter reduces DNA through affinity chromatography step. An enzymatic treatment is also utilized in the chromatography buffer wash to further degrade DNA that binds to the chromatography media. At the end of the purification processes, the amount of residual host cell DNA and its size distribution are determined using a quantitative PCR and a direct-labeling method, respectively. The two measures are key characteristics pertinent to the efficiency of the purification processes in reducing residual DNA-related risk, including the one caused by unmethylated CpG, which is described in the next section. CpG risk control is achieved by limiting both the amount and size of residual DNA in final dose. In this section, a method developed by Yang et al. (2015) is described. Through mechanistic modeling of DNA inactivation process using enzyme, Yang et al. (2015) linked the probability of immunogenic event DNA size and amount in the final product, both of which are risk factors. Such linkage enables the establishment of a simultaneous acceptance range for both factors such that product with DNA size and amount varying within the range has acceptable immunogenicity risk.

5.3.2.1 Risk of Residual Host Cell DNA

Biological products are often manufactured from cells. Therefore they often contain residual DNA from the host cells used in production. It is possible that the product may contain CpG motifs from the host cells. CpG motifs are short single-stranded synthetic DNA molecules containing a cytosine triphosphate deoxynucleotide and a guanine triphosphate deoxynucleotide. Unmethylated CpG motifs can act as immunostimulants as CpG motifs are considered pathogen-associated molecular patterns (PAMPs), and recognized by germline encoded receptors, also called pattern recognition receptors, such as the Toll-like receptors (TLRs) (Foged and Sundblad (2008)). Although CpG motifs are prevalent in microbial but not in vertebrate genomes, it is possible that residual DNA could contain immunostimulatory CpG motifs and may be immunostimulatory. In both preclinical and clinical studies, immune responses to CpG motifs used as either DNA vaccines or adjuvants have been reported (Klinman et al. (1997)). Also observed are anti-DNA antibodies (Al Arfaj et al. (2007), Bastian et al. (1985), Gilkeson et al. (1989), Karounos et al. (1988) , Pisetsky (1997), Stollar and Voss (1986)). These studies further demonstrate that the extent of immune response in animals is proportional to the amount of CpG in a plasmid and the ratio of CpG to all DNA present (Klinman et al. (1997), Kojima et al. (2002), Wang et al. (2012)). Therefore, residual DNA may have the potential to cause immunogenic reactions, and is a risk factor that needs to be carefully assessed.

5.3.2.2 Control Strategies

To mitigate the immunogenicity potential of residual DNA, it is necessary to estimate the immunogenicity risk due to CpG motifs. This includes estimation of severity and probability for CpG motifs to be present in the final product. Subsequently, the control strategy can be devised accordingly. Most recently Yang et al. (2015) developed a method through modeling the stochastic process of enzymatic degradation of residual DNA. A functional relationship is established between residual DNA and immunogenic response. Such linkage makes it possible to define ranges for both the amount and size of residual DNA in the final product such that the probability of inducing an unwanted immunogenic event is controlled at an acceptable level when the amount and size of DNA are within the ranges. To simplify our discussion, we assume that the host cell may potentially contain one CpG motif though development of the method does not require the assumption.

It is conceivable that by reducing the size and amount of residual DNA one may reduce the immunogenicity risk of CpG. Knowing it is impossible to degrade residual DNA to fragments of zero length or to make the final product free of residual DNA, control strategy should be centered on setting acceptable limits on these two critical characteristics of the residual DNA. Using the same mathematical notations as in Yang et al. (2015), we define X to be the number of intact CpG motifs in the final dose, and let θ_S and θ_U be the median size and average content (ng/dose) of residual DNA in the final dose, respectively. Since the overall immunogenicity risk due to CpG is tied up with number of doses used annually, we introduce N as the maximum annual number of doses. Furthermore, we let $\tilde{X}$ denote the numbers of intact CpG motif in the bulk product from which the final N doses of finished product are made. The acceptable ranges are defined as

$$A = \{\theta \equiv (\theta_S, \theta_U) : \text{Risk score} = S \times Pr[\tilde{X} \geq x_0 | \theta] < r_0\} \qquad (5.1)$$

where S is severity score of CpG, x_0 is number of intact CpG motifs sufficient to induce an immunogenic event, and r_0 is a pre-specified maximal acceptable risk. In other words, the acceptable ranges consist of combinations of median size and amount of residual DNA such that the probability for the annual bulk product to contain enough CpG motifs to induce an immunogenic event is bounded by a maximal acceptable risk r_0. The number x_0 can be either extracted from literature or empirically determined using animal models while r_0 can be determined based on regulatory expectation or requirement. Since the mean number of CpG motifs in the final dose depends on the parameter $\theta = (\theta_S, \theta_U)$, it is denoted as $\lambda_X(\theta)$. Yang et al. (2015) use a Poisson distribution $Poi(\lambda_X(\theta))$ to describe the number of intact CpG motifs in the final dose. Since the total number of intact CpG motifs in a bulk lot of the product $\tilde{X}$ is a sum of Poisson distributions, it also follows a Poisson distribution (Haight and Haight (1967)) with mean parameters being $N\lambda_X(\theta)$. That is,

$$Pr[\tilde{X} \geq x_0|\theta] = 1 - \sum_{i=0}^{x_0-1} \frac{[N\lambda_X(\theta)]^i e^{-N\lambda_X(\theta)}}{i!}.$$

The acceptable ranges in Equation 5.1 can be defined by

$$A = \left\{ \theta : S \times \left[1 - \sum_{i=0}^{x_0-1} \frac{[N\lambda_X(\theta)]^i e^{-N\lambda_X(\theta)}}{i!} \right] < r_0 \right\} \qquad (5.2)$$

To determine the range, it is necessary to explicit link parameter $\lambda_X(\theta)$ with θ. This is accomplished through modeling the process of enzymatic reaction intended to degrade residual DNA into finer pieces, rendering a small chance of having intact CpG in the final product. The control strategy is developed so that the overall risk defined as the product of severity score and probability of occurrence is maintained below an acceptance limit.

5.3.2.3 DNA Inactivation

To reduce the risk of residual DNA, several purification steps can be taken in production. One typical technique is filtration. The risk of immunogenicity can be further reduced by enzymatic degradation of DNA to the size below that of CpG motifs. The process is schematically displayed in Figure 5.3.3. Enzyme reduces DNA size by cleaving the phosphate ester bonds between two adjacent nucleotides. At the end of enzymatic reaction, a CpG motif remains either intact or fragmented. For example, the CpG sequence in Figure 5.6 is eventually disrupted by enzyme.

In the following section, linkage between the probability to have an acceptable number of intact CpG motifs and residual DNA size and amount in the final dose, and enzyme cutting efficiency characterized as the probability for enzyme to sever off the phosphate ester bond between two adjacent nucleotides is established. Such linkage makes possible the determination of the acceptable range in Equation 5.2.

5.3.2.4 Determination of Acceptance Range

The median size and amount of the residual DNA in the final product can be used to describe the efficiency of the process. Intuitively, the smaller the size and the less the amount of the residual DNA, the less likely the final dose would contain sufficient number of intact CpG motifs. To model the relationship between probability of having intact CpG motifs in the final product and DNA size and amount, additional notations are needed. Let M and m represent sizes of the host genome and CpG motifs size, and U and V the

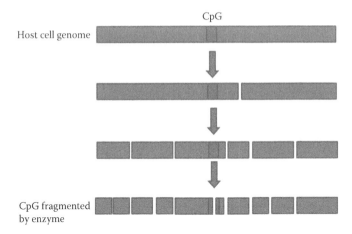

FIGURE 5.6
Diagram of DNA inactivation using enzyme. CpG sequence in the diagram is disrupted at the end of enzymatic reaction.

amount of residual DNA and total number of the CpG motifs (either intact or fragmented) in the final dose, respectively. Define d_O to the weight of CpG motif. Theoretically the quantity U/d_O represents the maximal number of CpG motifs a final dose may contain. Assuming that $V|U$ follows a binomial distribution $b(m/M, U/d_O)$ and $X|V$ follows $b(p_X, V)$ with p_X being the probability that a CpG remains intact after the enzymatic reaction, it can be readily shown that $E[V|U] = \frac{m}{M}(U/d_O)$ and $E[X|V] = p_X V$. Consequently, we obtain

$$\lambda_X(\theta) = E[X] = E_U\{E_V(E_X[X|V])|U\} = \left(\frac{p_X m E[U]}{d_O M}\right) = \frac{p_X m \theta_U}{d_O M}. \quad (5.3)$$

Yang et al. (2010) establish the link between the probability of getting a specific DNA sequence in a host cell genome and DNA cutting efficiency, characterized by the probability for enzyme to cut phosphate ester bond between two adjacent necleotides. Specifically, host cell genome and a specific DNA, say, CpG motifs, are expressed as

$$\Phi = B_1 c B_2 c \ldots c B_M, \quad \Omega = B_l c B_{l+1} c \ldots c B_{l+m-1}, \quad (5.4)$$

where B's and c are nucleotides and phosphate ester bond between two nucleotides, respectively, and l and m are integers. Define X_i as random variables that can take value either 0 or 1, with $P[X_i = 1] =$

$P[c_i$ is disrupted by the enzyme$] = 1 - P[X_i = 0] = p$. Assuming that X_is are IID following a Bernoulli distribution, the probability for the CpG motifs Ω not to be degraded by enzymatic reaction is

$$p_X = Pr[X_1 = X_2 \ldots = X_{m-1} = 0] = (1 - p)^{m-1}. \qquad (5.5)$$

Since the probability p for each phosphate ester bond to be severed depends on factors impacting enzymatic reaction process, some of which are known, and some are unknown, it is difficult to estimate experimentally. The method by Yang et al. (2010, 2015) provide an alternative way to estimate the probability. Let X' denote the size of a DNA segment randomly chosen from the reaction mix after a host genome is digested by enzyme. Such DNA segment takes the form of

$$B_{r+1}cB_{r+1}c \ldots cB_{r+X'} \qquad (5.6)$$

where r is an integer. Note that the size of the above DNA segment is the same as the number of failed attempts made by the enzyme at cutting through the bonds c's before it successfully disrupts the bonds c right after nucleotide $B_{r+X'}$. Yang et al. Yang et al. (2010) use a geometric distribution to describe X'. Thus,

$$Pr[X' = k] = (1 - p)^{k-1}p, \ k = 1, 2, \ldots, M - 1. \qquad (5.7)$$

Note that the theoretical median of X' is given by

$$\theta_S = -\frac{\log 2}{\log(1 - p)}. \qquad (5.8)$$

A relationship between enzyme cutting efficiency p and the median size of residual DNA is established through (5.8).

Combining (5.3), (5.5) and (5.8), we obtain

$$\lambda_X(\theta) = 2^{-(m-1)/\theta_S} \frac{m}{d_O M} \theta_U, \qquad (5.9)$$

The above equation indicates that the average number of intact CpG in the final dose is a function of the size of host genome, the size of CpG motif, and the size and amount of CpG motifs in the final dose. Since the risk score of getting at least x_0 number intact CpG in bulk materials in 5.1 is a monotonically decreasing function, it can be controlled by limiting below certain levels, which in turn can be accomplished by controlling both the size and amount of residual DNA.

5.3.2.5 Numerical Calculations

We illustrate the use of the method developed in the previous sections to establish the control strategies of immunogenic risk due to CpG motifs. It is assumed that severity of immunogenicity caused by CpG motifs is very high,

TABLE 5.4
Parameter values needed for design of control strategy

Parameter	Description	Value
m	Size of unmytholated CpG motif	100 bp
M	Size of host genome	2.41×10^9 bp
A	Amount of CpG motifs needed to induce an immunogenic event	$9.6\mu g$
N	Annual number of doses used	5×10^7

thus has a value of 9 per Table 5.2. The haploid genome size of the MDCK cell is determined to be 2.41×10^9 bp. It is of interest to estimate the probability of getting an immunogenic event for various combinations of DNA size and amount $\theta = (\theta_S, \theta_U)$, more specifically, to determine the following acceptable ranges of size and amount of residual DNA in final product in 5.2. To that end, we first need to estimate x_0, the number of intact CpG motif needed to induce an immonogenic event. It is further assumed that it requires 9.6 μg CpG motifs to induce an immunogenic event and that CpG motif of interest has a size of 100. The above assumptions are summarized in Table 5.4.

Estimates of the molecular weights (MW) for dA, dC, dT, and dG are 313.2, 289.2, 304.2, and 329.2, respectively. So for a 100 bp DNA, the MW is $100/2 \times (313.2 + 289.2 + 304.2 + 329.2) = 61790$ g/mol. Thus 9.6 $\mu g/61790$ g/mol=$1.55 \times 10^{-4}\mu$ mole=1.55×10^{-10} mole. Note that 1 mole has 6.022×10^{23} molecules, so 1.55×10^{-10} mole has $1.55 \times 10^{-10} \times 6.022 \times 10^{23} = 9.67 \times 10^{13}$ molecules of CpG motifs. In other words,

$$x_0 = 9.67 \times 10^{13} \text{ molecules of CpG motifs.} \qquad (5.10)$$

We assume that potentially a maximum of 50 million doses can be produced annually ($N = 5 \times 10^7$). A plot of the probability function $Pr[\tilde{X} \geq x_0|\theta]$ used to define the acceptable ranges is constructed and displayed in Figure 5.7. The plot depicts the risk of having one immunogenic event out of the total number of 50 million doses produced for various combinations of median DNA size and amount of DNA in the final dose. For example, for $\theta = (200bp, 10ng)$ which are regulatory limits for residual DNA in the final dose, the corresponding probability of having at least one immunogenicity event is calculated to be less than 10^{-15}. Setting r_0, the pre-specified maximal risk in 5.1, at 10^{-15}, the acceptable ranges of residual DNA size and amount correspond to the shaded area on the plane of $\theta = (\theta_S, \theta_U)$ in Figure 5.8.

Application of the model requires some prior knowledge. For example, the amount of CpG motifs that can induce an immunogenic event is a required quantity. In practice, an estimate of this quantity from clinical studies is not feasible due to ethical concerns. Animal models can be used as surrogates. As pointed out by many researchers, animal models in general have limited predictive capability for immunogenicity in humans. However, the immunogenic

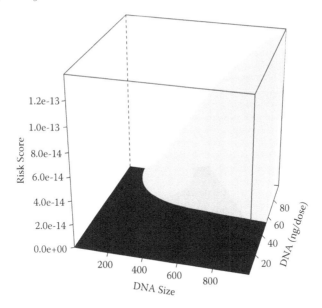

FIGURE 5.7
Plot of risk score of having an immunogenic event caused by unmethylated CpG motifs, based on annual use of 50 million doses of the product.

amount of CpG motifs estimated from animal studies is likely a conservative estimation. Therefore, probability of occurrence estimated based on the animal model is also likely over-estimating the real probability of immunogenicity event. In this sense, it can be directly used in risk assessment. The example presented in this section is a demonstration that statistical modeling can be effectively utilized to understand immunogenic risk, and serve as a basis for establishing control strategies.

5.4   Biomarkers for Immunogenicity

As previously discussed, some patient's characteristics predispose the subjects to have an immunogenic response to some biological therapies. One way to mitigate immunogenicity risk is to segment the patient population so that the subset that is less prone to adverse immune reaction is identified. This subpopulation will be the target population during clinical development. Some biomarkers have been identified as possible indicators that a patient may be at risk of an immunogenic response. For example, unusually high and persisting levels of neutralizing antibodies are indicative of immunogenicity, and

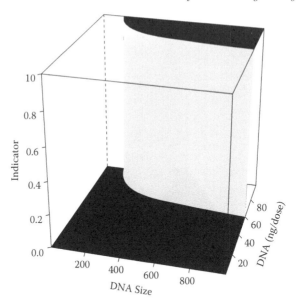

FIGURE 5.8
Acceptable range (dark area at the bottom of the plot) of DNA size and amount in final dose for a therapeutic protein with a maximal risk no more than 10^{-15}, assuming that maximally 50 million doses of the product are produced and used. The z-axis is values of an indicator function with values 0 and 1 corresponding to acceptable and unacceptable level of immunogenicity risk (risk score $\leq 10^{-15}$), respectively.

may be used to exclude high risk patients from clinical studies. However, since factors that impact immunogenicity are rarely independent, application of a univariate marker is inadequate to differentiate one group of subjects from another. For example, we assume that two risk factors X and Y are associated with product immunogenicity. It is also assumed that measurements of X and Y are taken for two groups of patients called A and B, one group having ADA responses (shown in diamond, in Figure 5.9) and the other not having ADA responses (shown in square, in Figure 5.9). Examination of the data reveals that for immunogenic group A, the measurements of $X(Y)$ tends to be lower(higher) than that of group B. However, if the patients are classified as at risk for the development of an immunogenic response or not at risk based on checking X and Y against their respective cut-off points x_0 and y_0, there are no cut-off values (x_0, y_0) that render complete separation of the two groups. Several alternative methods, all multivariate in nature, can overcome the drawback of the above approach. One is linear discriminant analysis (LDA) and other is principal component analysis (PCA).

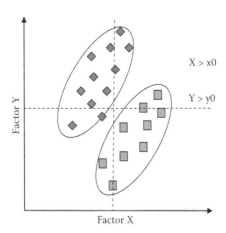

FIGURE 5.9

Insufficiency of individual or combined assessment of factors X and Y in predicting immunogenic risk: neither factor X, factor Y, nor their combination.

Linear discriminant analysis is a statistical method that attempts to separate two or more classes of objects, based on a linear combination of measured characteristics of the objects. The resulting combination is used as a classifier to assign group membership for each new object. In the above example, it is evident that a linear combination of X and Y can result in complete separation between groups A and B (see Figure 5.10). As there is variability associated with each measurement, complete separation of groups is impossible, and the performance of LDA needs to be validated through independent data.

A closely related technique is principal component analysis. Common to both methods is identification of linear combinations of the risk factors to best describe data. While LDA focuses on modeling differences between groups, PCA, looks for a few linear combinations (commonly referred to as principal components) to explain variability in data. .

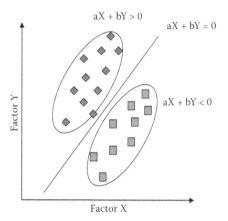

FIGURE 5.10
A linear combination of the two factors can clearly differentiate Group A from Group B.

In this section, various statistical methods for identifying potential immunogenicity biomarkers for patient segmentation are discussed. In addition to the aforesaid LDA and PCA methods, other clustering methods and predictive models are introduced. Also included in this section are general strategies for immunogenicity biomarker discovery, and cross-validation of statistical models for patient segmentation. Several examples are used to illustrate some of the methods introduced.

5.4.1 General Strategies

An immunogenicity biomarker is a measurable indicator of an immunogenic risk. As previously discussed, it can be any of the product-intrinsic factors, product-extrinsic factors, patient-related characteristics, or a combination of factors. Additionally, a single factor, deemed to be not predictive of immunogenicity, may be a good biomarker when used in combination with others factors. Therefore, in a broad sense, an immunogenicity biomarker can be a combination of factors. To account for such inter-dependence, appropriate statistical methods need to be used.

As biomarkers used for mitigating immunogenicity risk are intended to identify a patient population that is less likely to have immunogenic responses for participation in a clinical trial, ideally the smaller the number of biomarkers is, the more efficient and less costly the trials are. Consequently, a general biomarker strategy should be oriented toward utilization of a smaller set of biomarkers to maximally predict immune response. This is also driven by statistical considerations. Early clinical trials usually consist of a small number of subjects. In such cases, a statistical model used for patient selection tends to be over-fitted, making it sensitive to perturbations of the biomarkers in the model. Consequently, early clinical trial models may not be suitable for classifying future patients.

To limit the number of biomarkers that enter the prediction model, the first step is to use clustering methods to put biomarkers into groups. The dimension of each of the groups can be further reduced through PCA (see Section 5.4.3). Each group represented by either its principal components or mean value, can be used as a predictor in a discriminant analysis model (refer to Section 5.4.4).

5.4.2 Clustering Methods

The primary aim of clustering analysis is to group immunogenicity risk factors into a small number of groups. Risk factors in the same group are similar by certain statistical measures. A natural grouping for immunogenicity risk factors is to categorize them into 3 groups which would be the product-intrinsic factors, product-extrinsic factors, and patient-related characteristics. In this section, two methods, K-means clustering and hierarchical clustering, are discussed and illustrated with an example. The methods introduced are usually referred to as unsupervised clustering as they do not rely on the knowledge of the immunogenicity status (immune responder versus non-responder) of patients.

5.4.2.1 K-Means Clustering

K-means clustering was first proposed by MacQueen (1967). The method is designed to classify p factors into k clusters (groups) where K is the only input parameter required. A large K allows for forming small groups containing a number of tightly related biomarkers; while a small K only allows for forming large groups. The number k is an ancillary parameter and may be initially selected based on subject knowledge. For example, $K=3$ may correspond to the natural grouping of immunogenicity risk factors.

A data set used for immunogenicity biomarker identification usually consists of risk factor measurements from a certain number of samples(subjects). Mathematically, it can be expressed as $\{x_1, x_2, ..., x_p\}$, where p is the total number of risk factors, n is the number of samples, and x_i is the measurements of the ith risk factor for all n samples. x_i represents one data point in an n dimensional space. As discussed before, during early clinical development it is common that $p > n$. We denote μ_k as the center of the kth cluster, which is usually unknown, but can be estimated through an iterative process. The objective of the K-means clustering method is to find the center of each cluster, $\{C_1, C_2, ..., C_K\}$ that minimizes the total within cluster sum of squares

$$\sum_{k=1}^{K} \sum_{x_i \in C_k} \|x_i - \mu_k\|^2 \tag{5.11}$$

The initial K center points are randomly generated, then each of the p biomarkers is assigned to the group which has the shortest distance to its group center. After all the biomarkers have been assigned, the centers are re-calculated. All the biomarkers are re-assigned using the new centers until the assignments no longer change. Since the initial centers may not be the same each time one runs the analysis, the resulting K clusters may be different as well. Note that the above method uses the Euclidean distance as the similarity measure. Alternatively, the Euclidean distance can be replaced by the correlation measure. If the correlation measure is used, measurements of each risk factor x_i need to be standardized first before applying this clustering method. Denote $x_i = (x_{i,1}, \ldots, x_{i,n})$, the standardized measurements $\{y_1, y_2, ..., y_p\}$ are all centered at 0 with standard deviation 1.

$$y_{i,g} = \frac{x_{i,g} - \bar{x}_i}{\sqrt{\frac{\sum_{g=1}^{n}(x_{i,g} - \bar{x}_i)^2}{n-1}}} \tag{5.12}$$

The correlation between the new variables $y_{l,m}$ becomes

$$cor(y_l, y_m) = \frac{\sum_g (x_{l,g} - \bar{x}_l)(x_{m,g} - \bar{x}_m)}{\sqrt{\sum_g (x_{l,g} - \bar{x}_l)^2}\sqrt{\sum_g (x_{m,g} - \bar{x}_m)^2}} \tag{5.13}$$

$$= 1 - \frac{1}{2}\sum_g (y_{l,g} - y_{m,g})^2 \tag{5.14}$$

5.4.2.2 Hierarchical Clustering

In hierarchical clustering (HC), one is not limited to Euclidean distance or correlation measures. HC has additional distance measures such as Manhattan distance and maximum distance. The method starts to form groups by merging two biomarkers that have the shortest distance. The distances between this group of biomarkers with other biomarkers or biomarker groups are re-calculated using a predefined linkage criterion. A linkage criterion determines the distance between two groups of biomarkers. For example, the maximum linkage between two groups of biomarkers is the maximum distance of all pairs of biomarkers in the two groups; minimum linkage is the minimum distance of all pairs of biomarkers; centroid linkage is the distance between the centers of two clusters; and the average linkage is the average distances of all pairs of the biomarkers. Centroid linkage and average linkage are used more often than other linkage methods in practice.

The result of HC is presented as a dendrogram. The biomarkers are clustered by cutting the branches at different heights (distances). Contrary to K-means clustering, some biomarkers may not be clustered. Only those biomarkers with heights below the pre-chosen threshold are clustered and the remaining biomarkers are not clustered. By adjusting the height threshold, one can control the number and size of clusters. To illustrate how these two clustering methods perform in practice, we simulate a data set with 100 biomarkers collected from 40 samples.

5.4.2.3 Comparison of Clustering by K-Means and HC Using Simulated Data

We use a simulated data set to illustrate the use of clustering methods discussed above. The data include measurements of 100 risk factors from 40 samples. Of the 40 samples, 20 samples are immunogenicity true-positive and 20 samples are immunogenicity true-negative. The risk factors are simulated in such a way that twelve risk factors correlate with the immunogenicity status as shown in Figure 5.11. It means that the immune responders have higher values for these 12 risk factors than those who are non-immune responders. In addition, 25 risk factors are simulated so that they are weakly correlated with the immunogenicity status and the rest 63 factors are not correlated with immunogenicity status. The simulated data is visualized using a heat map plot in Figure 5.11.

The HC and K-means results are shown in Figure 5.12. The HC clustering is performed with thresholds set at 0.5 and 0.8, and the K-means clustering is performed assuming there are 3 clusters. It can be seen that the K-means method is able to identify the two relevant clusters correctly. HC with a 0.5 threshold captures most of the members in the two clusters, but at 0.8 threshold, the two clusters are merged together. It is evident that the hierarchical clustering method highly relies on selecting an appropriate threshold. When the threshold is too high or too low, the clusters are not well defined. However, Zhang and Horvath (2005) have developed a dynamic cluster detection method which gives tremendous help to automate searching for clusters.

5.4.2.4 Principal Component Analysis

Principal component analysis (PCA) is a classic multivariate analysis tool, primarily used for dimension reduction. However, it is often found useful to confirm a clustering result. PCA rotates the data matrix in the high dimensional space of risk factors such that the first component represents the most variant direction; the second orthogonal component represents the second most variant direction, and so on. The components are typically expressed as linear combinations of risk factors with the first component containing the

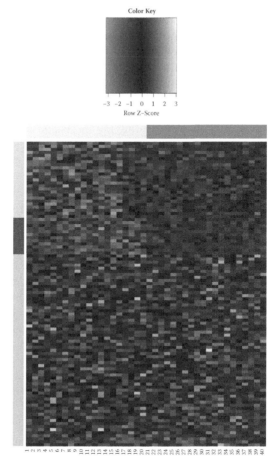

FIGURE 5.11
A simulated data set with 100 risk factors from 40 samples. The x-axis lists the samples and the y-axis displays the risk factors.

information of the most variant data, and the last component containing the information of the least variant data. Usually, the first few components are selected to represent the data, resulting in reduction of data dimension. The selected components can be used as predictors in discriminant analysis models such as those discussed in the next section.

For clustering purpose, it is prudent that all the risk factor measurements are normalized to mean=0 and variance=1 before the analysis. This is because different risk factors may be measured at different scales. Data normalization gives each risk factor equal weight in the analysis. When the first few principle components contain nearly all the information in the data, clusters often

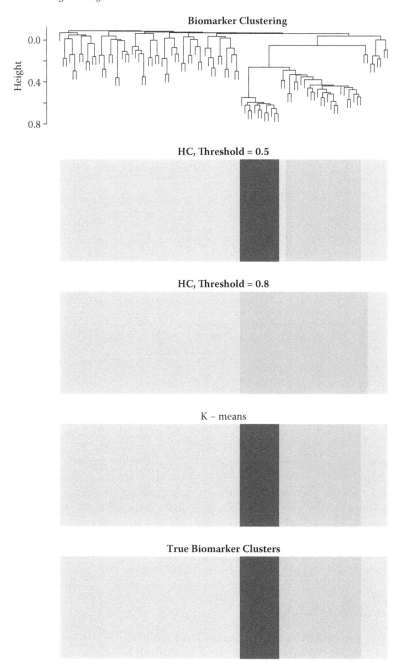

FIGURE 5.12

Comparing hierarchical clustering with K-means clustering methods. The thresholds used for HC method are 0.5 and 0.8 and $K=3$ clusters are used for K-means clustering method.

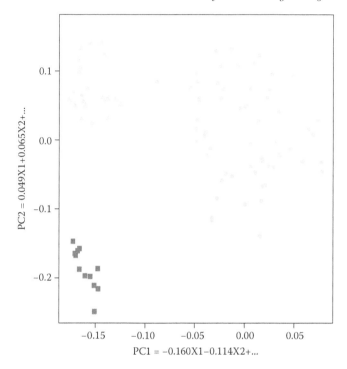

FIGURE 5.13
Principal component analysis of the simulated biomarker data. Visualization uses the first two principal vectors.

become self-evident when being projected to the subspace defined by these principal components.

Figure 5.13 shows the simulated risk factor data projected to the two dimensional space defined by the first two principal components. All three risk factor clusters are clearly separated. However, without knowing the clusters *a priori*, trying to define the clusters based on the projected data visualization is a subjective practice and we do not suggest using PCA as a primary tool for cluster detection.

5.4.3   Prediction Models

Clustering analysis and PCA help to reduce large dimensional risk factor data into smaller risk factor groups. Each of these groups can be either represented by the group mean or by the first principal component. Dimension reduction makes building predictive models possible. Predictive models are also known as statistical classifiers, which are used to segment patients into immune response and non-immune response groups. Three commonly used predictive models are the logistic regression model, linear discriminant analysis (LDA) model, and K-Nearest Neighbors (KNN). The logistic regression model and LDA are parametric methods while the KNN method is nonparametric.

5.4.3.1 Logistic Regression Model

For p biomarkers $X = \{X_1, X_2, ..., X_p\}_{n \times p}$, the logistic regression model can be written as

$$Pr(Positive|X) = \frac{\exp(\beta_0 + \beta^T X)}{1 + \exp(\beta_0 + \beta^T X)} \tag{5.15}$$

$$Pr(Negative|X) = \frac{1}{1 + \exp(\beta_0 + \beta^T X)} \tag{5.16}$$

This method uses the logistic function of the linear combination of the biomarkers to estimate the probability of positive or negative immunogenicity. After all the parameters $\{\hat{\beta}_0, \hat{\beta}\}$ are properly estimated, for a new sample with biomarker profile X_{new}, one can classify it to immunogenicity positive group if $\hat{\beta}_0 + \hat{\beta}^T X_{new} > 0$.

The decision boundary for a logistic regression model is a hyperplane, which is a point when there is one biomarker and a straight line when there are two biomarkers.

One serious drawback of the logistic regression method is multi-collinearity between biomarkers. When it happens, the parameter estimations become inaccurate. Although parameter selection procedures may help reducing the multi-collinearity effects by reducing the number of biomarkers in the prediction model, important biologically meaningful biomarkers may get un-selected in the process, which can be a dilemma one has to face in practice.

5.4.3.2 *K*-Nearest Neighbors (KNN)

The KNN method calculates the distance of a new sample to all the samples in the training sets. Thus, KNN is one of the simplest yet most flexible model, as it only has a single parameter that may or may not need to be estimated. The new sample is classified to the immunogenicity-positive group if the majority of the K-nearest samples are in the immunogenicity-positive group. The method can be seen as a democratic voting of the K-selected representatives. It is prudent to avoid selecting an even number of K because it may happen that the new sample cannot be classified to either group when votes are tied. Unlike other model based classifiers, the KNN method does not need to estimate parameters. Since the classification of a new sample depends only on the K-nearest training samples, the training samples farther from the new sample have no influence on the classification. The resulting decision boundary is flexible, adjusting itself according to the local sample compositions.

5.4.3.3 Linear Discriminant Analysis (LDA)

LDA assumes that the probability densities of the risk factors are normally distributed for both immunogenicity-positive and immunogenicity-negative samples. The method aims at finding the optimal linear combination of risk factors such that the immunogenicity-positive and immunogenicity-negative samples are best separated. Let W be the coefficients of a linear combination of all risk factors y. Thus W is a vector of n dimension. W can be determined such that the ratio of within class variation and between class variation of the linear combination of the risk factor is minimized.

$$\underset{W}{\mathrm{argmin}}\, \frac{W^{'} S_{within} W}{W^{'} S_{between} W} \tag{5.17}$$

In the following, we use a simulated example to illustrate the utility of LDA. In this example, previous studies identified aggregation and deamination as two potential biomarkers to segment patients. Five hundred samples are simulated from bivariate normal distributions for immunogenicity-positive and immunogenicity-negative group. The circle and triangle dots in Figure 5.14 represent immunogenicity-positive/-negative groups. The values of the two risk factors are bounded within (-3, 3); one group is centered at (-2, -2) and the other group is centered at (2, 2); the two groups have a common covariance matrix

$$\Sigma = \begin{bmatrix} 2 & 0.1 \\ 0.1 & 2 \end{bmatrix}$$

The linear combinations of aggregation and deamination were created using $W_1 = (1, 0), W_2 = (0, 1), W_3 = (0.707, 0.707), W_4 = (-0.707, 0.707)$, resulting in four data sets. The data sets are plotted in Figure 5.15. Based on this analysis, the linear combination with the coefficients $W_3 = (0.707, 0.707)$ rendered the biggest separations between immunogenicity-positive and immunogenicity-negative groups. The two groups are completely indistinguishable when $W_4 = (-0.707, 0.707)$ is used to construct the linear combination.

In general, after the optimal linear combination is determined, a classification rule can be developed based on the distance of the linear combination of a new sample, and the center points of the clusters that were calculated from the linear combination. The sample is classified to immunogenicity-positive group if it is closer to its group center and vice versa for the immunogenicity-negative group.

However, calculating W involves calculating the inverse of the covariance matrix, Σ^{-1}. This is not an issue when the number of samples is greater than the number of biomarkers. However, when the number of biomarkers is greater than the number of samples, Σ is a singular matrix and its inverse is not available. In such cases, the LDA method cannot be applied. One remedy as proposed by Dudoit et al. (2002) is to only use the diagonal elements of

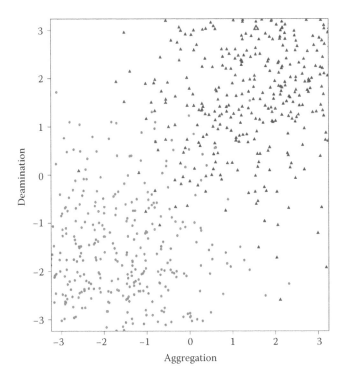

FIGURE 5.14
Simulated segregation of 500 samples into immunogenicity-positive and immunogenicity-negative groups. The values of the two risk factors are standardized such that they are contained with (-3,3). Circle and triangle dots correspond to immunogenicity-positive and immunogenicity-negative groups, respectively.

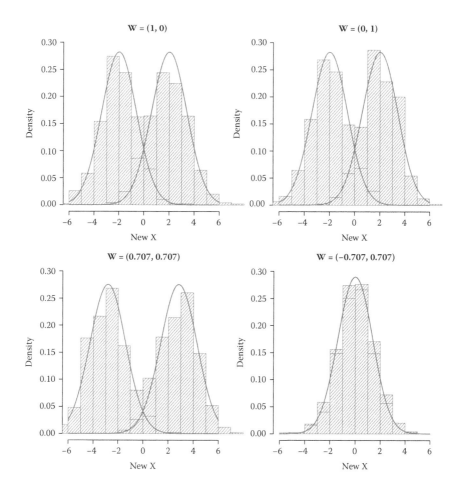

FIGURE 5.15
Immunogenicity distributions based on $W_1 = (1,0), W_2 = (0,1), W_3 = (0.707, 0.707), W_4 = (-0.707, 0.707)$.

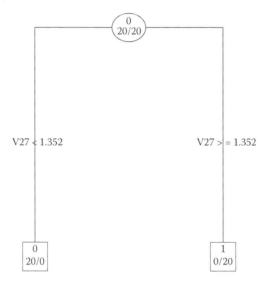

FIGURE 5.16
Classification of the simulated 100 biomarker data using rpart() function.

the covariance matrix; this new method is called diagonal linear discriminant analysis (DLDA). DLDA actually performs better than LDA and other more complicated methods in real data analysis.

5.4.3.4 Classification Tree and Random Forest Methods

Random Forest(RF) has gained much popularity in recent decades. As the name suggests, the RF is an ensemble of classification trees. The tree method first finds one risk factor that best partitions immunogenicity-positive and immunogenicity-negative samples. Through recursive partitioning, one can arrive at a node in the end that no further partition is possible. The tree itself represents a classification rule. Figure 5.16 shows a simple classification result using the simulated data in section 5.4.2.2. The risk factor $V27$ perfectly partitions the samples to immunogenicity-positive and immunogenicity-negative groups. When $V27 < 1.352$, all 20 samples are immunogenicity-negative; when $V27 \geq 1.352$, all 20 samples are immunogenicity-positive.

Such clear separation between different groups seldom happens in practice. Due to the large number of risk factors, unrelated risk factors may appear to be predictive in the training set but prove to be unreliable in independent data sets. Since tree methods tend to over-fit a data set (especially when $p > n$), the prediction using tree method is often unstable. One tree may be unstable, but an ensemble of many trees would solve the stability problem. The random forest method uses a part of the training data to select biomarkers and build tree classifiers, and use the remaining of the training data (oob:out-of-bag) to assess classification error and variable importance. A future sample is classified according to the vote of all the trees.

RF method can also be used to do biomarker selection. Since not all biomarkers will be selected in each tree classifier, those biomarkers selected more frequently can be deemed as more important. It should be easy to device a method that selects biomarkers based on their frequency of appearing in tree classifiers and weighted by their tandem orders.

5.4.3.5   Cross Validation and Bagging

Cross validation method is used to access the performance of a proposed statistical method in an independent data set. It divides n samples into k groups and uses $\frac{(k-1)n}{k}$ samples to train the predictive model and use the remaining $\frac{n}{k}$ samples as a validation set to examine the predictive accuracy. For binary outcome like immunogenicity presence, one can use C-index as a measure of concordance between the predicted outcome and the observed outcome in the validation set. Leaving-one-out cross validation is also called Jackknife. Other popular choices are leave N/2 out and leave N/3 out. One can report the distribution of C-index (`rcorr.cens()` function in R) as the performance of the statistical model for one specific data set. To predict the immunogenicity status of new samples, one can use an ensemble of all models and take the average prediction as the final result.

Bagging is an abbreviation of Bootstrap aggregating using statistical classification methods. Most of the time, we are limited to small sample sizes and it is impractical to infer the distribution of the population. One idea is to resample (bootstrapping) the data with replacement to assess the sampling variation. For each bootstrap sample, one can apply the interested predictive method and an ensemble of all the predictors can be the final predictor for the data set.

5.4.3.6   Simple Is a Virtue

The data set one uses to build a classification model is called a training set. The training set data has two training purposes. The first is to estimate the parameters of the classification model. Secondly it is to evaluate the predictive errors, which is important when one needs to compare all the classification models and select one for the future clinical studies. In a certain sense, training data set itself is more critical than the predictor models. If the quality of the training data is compromised, no matter how appropriate the predictor model is, it can't predict the immunogenicity responses of candidate patients.

An ideal training set should be representative and balanced, and comes from a well-thought-out design. Representativeness means that the training samples should be representative of the target patient population. Balanced means that the immunogenicity-positive samples and the immunogenicity-negative samples in the training set should be roughly the same. For a large study that takes a long time to finish, day-to-day variation, batch-to-batch variation, and operator-to-operator variation should be considered ahead and be reflected in the design accordingly.

Predictive models are only as good as the data. When the data are good, most predictive methods, both simple and complicated, should all work well. We prefer simple methods like KNN and DLDA, as they have fewer procedural issues to deal with and it is easier to interpret the results as well.

5.5 Concluding Remarks

Immunogenicity risk control is an integral part of clinical development of therapeutic proteins. The control strategy starts with criticality determination of potential risk factors. Such assessment relies on prior knowledge, and historical and current data. The criticality estimation serves as the basis for finding risk factors that are likely to have major impact on product safety and efficacy. Following the identification of risk factors, control strategies are developed. Of note is that immunogenicity control is multi-faceted, including selection of less immunogenic candidate proteins for clinical development, enhanced ADA monitoring plan, control of both product- and process-related risk factors through acceptance testing and specifications, accounting for interdependence among risk factors, and using immunogenicity biomarkers/diagnostic indices as inclusion/exclusion criteria for patient selection in clinical trials. It is conceivable that the elements of an immunogenicity control strategy evolve as the protein progresses from one stage of drug development to another. Thus immunogenicity control strategy should be developed with a view of product lifecycle and close collaboration among statisticians, scientists, and clinicians is critical to adjust the control strategy effectively.

6

Computational Tools for Immunogenicity Analysis

In this chapter,we use examples in R and SAS languages to illustrate how to conduct the various analyses discussed throughout this book.

6.1 Read Data into R

Reading data into the R environment is the first step of the analysis and there are many ways to do it. For a small data set, the simplest way is to read directly from the clipboard using *read.table()* function.

```
x=read.table("clipboard", header=F)
```

read.table() function reads data organized in a tab delimited text file (*.txt*). *read.csv()* function reads data organized in a comma delimited file (*.csv*). If the data is organized in an Excel *.xlsx* file with multiple sheets, one has to rely on the *read.xlsx()* function in the xlsx package. *readColumns()* is a slightly complicated alternative to read *.xlsx* file.

```
x=read.xlsx(file,which_sheet,which_rows,which_columns)
```

For many analyses, it is easier to work with a data frame than a data list in R. So, after the data is read into the R environment, it is necessary to check the data type.

```
is.list(x)         # check if the data is a list object
is.data.frame(x)   # check if the data is a data.frame object
x=as.data.frame(x) # coerce the data to a data.frame objet
```

6.2   ADA Assay and Cut Point

6.2.1   ADA Assay Development

The *drm* function in drc package can be used for calibration curve fitting. Assume that response-concentration data are stored in a data.frame called res_conc in which the variable donor_id is a factor, distinguishing data from different donors.

```
library(drc)
curve.fit<-drm(signal~concentration,data=res_conc,fct=LL.4(),
          curveid=donor_id)
```

In function *drm*, the parameter *fct* specifies which curve to fit. In this case, the four-parameter log-logistic *LL.4()* in model (2.2) is used.

Random-effect calibration curve can be fitted using function *nlme* in the nlme package.

```
random.curve.fit<-
  nlme(signal ~ c+(d-c)/(1+exp(b*(log(concentration)-log(e)))),
  data = res_conc, weights=varPower(),
  groups=~donor_id,
  fixed = b + c + d + e ~ 1,
  random = pdDiag(b + c + d + e~ 1),
  start = c(b = stv[1], c = stv[2], d = stv[3], e = stv[4]))
```

In this model, all the curve parameters b, c, d, e are assumed to be random from the donor population and normally distributed. The *random* parameter in *nlme* function assumes that b, c, d, e are independent. *start* uses the initial values for these curve parameters which needs to be specified. The vector stv are the initial values from the *drm* output. The *weights* parameter is optional but very flexible and can take a variance function form such as those mentioned for model (2.5).

The function *lme* in package **nlme** and *lmer* in package **lme4** can be used for nested ANOVA analysis. For data in a structure as in Figure 2.3,

```
library(nlme)
model1<-lme(signal~1, random=~1|analyst/day,data=yourdata)
summary(model1)
```

or

```
library(lme4)
model2<-lmer(signal~1+(1|analyst/day),data=yourdata)
summary(model2)
```

As can be seen, the specification of random part in *lme* and *lmer* is similar. If there is additional nested layer (factor), it can be added to the model in a similar way. To extract the variance components, use function *VarCorr*, e.g., VarCorr(model1).

To generate design table for various types of experimental designs, the JMP DOE module, among other DOE softwares, is a convenient tool with user-friendly GUI and very detailed technical documentation. In R, the function *FrF2* in package **FrF2** implements regular fractional factorial 2-level designs. The code to generate a design similar to Table 2.2 is:

```
library(FrF2)
plan <- FrF2(nruns = 16, nfactors = 5)
summary(plan)
```

The parameter **ncenter** can be used to add center design points to the factorial design to test possible curvature.

The function *pb* generates Plackett–Burman designs and in some cases other screening designs in run numbers that are a multiple of 4. For example,

```
library(FrF2)
pb.plan<-pb(nruns=12)
summary(pb.plan)
```

The total number of runs (**nruns**) has to be specified first instead of number of factors. By default, the **nfactors** parameter in *pb* function is set to be nruns-1.

The functions *ccd* and *bbd* in package rsm are available to generate standard response surface designs. For example, to generate a Box–Behnken design with 3 factors and 4 central points, the R code is:

```
library(rms)
bbd.design<-bbd(3, n0=4)
```

To generate a central composite design (CCD), call the following code:

```
library(rms)
ccd.design<-ccd(3, n0=c(4,6),alpha = "spherical")
```

Note that the parameter n0 requires a vector of two numbers, namely, the number of central points and the number of axial points. The parameter alpha asks which type of CCD is intended. It has several options such as "orthogonal, spherical, rotatable, and faces" with the default one is "orthogonal". The rsm package also has a function *ccd.pick* for choosing an optimal design from nonstandard designs. The interested readers should consult the package help documentation for details including the example of sequential optimization strategy from fractional factorial design. In JMP, the "response surface design" window in the DOE module can generate these standard response surface designs very conveniently. It also generates design tables, which can be analyzed once the experimental data are obtained.

Analysis of split-plot design is different from that of completely randomized design as shown in Table 2.4. Although both analyses can be conducted using the function *aov*, the model specification is very different as shown in the following code.

```
data <- matrix(c(1,360,1,67,1,360,2,73,
                 1,360,3,83,1,360,4,89,
                 2,370,1,65,2,370,2,91,
                 2,370,3,87,2,370,4,86,
                 3,380,1,155,3,380,2,127,
                 3,380,3,147,3,380,4,212,
                 4,380,1,108,4,380,2,100,
                 4,380,3,90,4,380,4,153,
                 5,370,1,140, 5,370,2,142,
                 5,370,3,121,5,370,4,150,
                 6,360,1,33,6,360,2,8,
                 6,360,3,46,6,360,4,54),byrow=T,ncol=4)
Block <- factor(data[,1])
Temp <- factor(data[,2])
Coat <- factor(data[,3])
## complete randomized design
aov.fit1 <- aov(data[,4] ~ Temp + Coat + Temp*Coat)
```

```
summary(aov.fit1)
## split-plot design
aov2.fit2 <- aov(data[,4] ~ Temp + Coat + Temp*Coat
            + Error(Block/Coat))
summary(aov2.fit2)
```

In the analysis of split-plot design, the `Error` term specifies the whole plot and subplot.

6.2.2 Implementation of White Paper Approach

In this subsection, we will demonstrate the implementation of Shankar et al.'s (Shankar et al., 2008) approach for cut point determination as described in section 3.3.

Assuming that x is a generic vector representing donors' signals or the average signals across the runs, the *boxcox* function in `MASS` package can be used to find the optimal transformation.

```
library(MASS)
boxcox(x~1,lambda=c(-3,3,0.1))
```

The *boxcox* function essentially finds the optimal λ by maximizing the likelihood on the grid within the range $[-3, 3]$ as specified by the user. As shown in the Figure 6.1 below, the function *boxcox* generates a plot by providing the 95% confidence interval for the optimal λ.

The skewness of a vector x characterizes the skewness of the distribution and defined as $E(X - \mu)^3/\sigma^3$. One can calculate the skewness of vector x by writing a simple function *skewness*:

```
skewness<-function(x){
m3<-sum((x-mean(x))^3)/length(x)
s3<-sd(x)^3
m3/s3 }
skewness(x)
```

Right-sknewed distribution has skewness greater than 0 and left-skewed distribution has skewness less than 0.

The simplest way to check normality assumption is the quantile-quantile (QQ) plot. This plots the ranked samples x against the same number of ranked quantiles taken from the normal distribution. If the data is normally distributed, these pair-wise dots will be along the straight line tightly as shown in Figure 6.2.

```
qqnorm(x)
qqline(x)
```

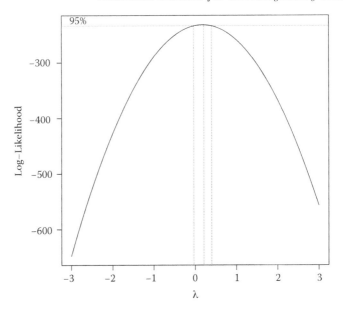

FIGURE 6.1
Example of finding optimal Box–Cox transformation.

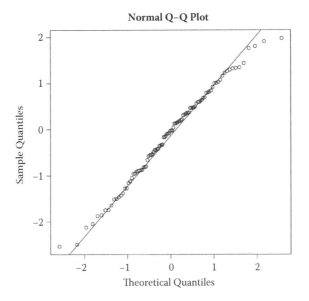

FIGURE 6.2
Example of QQ plot.

There are many formal tests available to test for the normality assumption, among which, the Shapiro–Wilk test is a popular one due to its superior power.

```
shapiro.test(x)
```

A p-value greater than 0.05 indicates that the data did not violate the assumption of normality.

The Box-plot method for outlier removal is based on the so-called inter-quartile range (IQR). Any data value below $Q_1 - k \times IQR$ or above $Q_3 + k \times IQR$ is considered a (suspected) outlier, where Q_1 and Q_3 are the first and third quartiles, respectively.

```
Lower_bound<-quantile(x,0.25)-k*IQR(x)
Upper_bound<-quantile(x,0.75)+k*IQR(x)
outliers<-x[x<Lower_bound | x> Upper_bound]
```

where k typically takes 1.5 or 3. Note that in R, quantile definitions is not unique. One can get details of these definitions by call *help(quantile)*. To compare the results from JMP or SAS, one should be aware of the definition discrepancy and choose the correct one.

To compare the run means and variances, the raw signals/responses of donors should be organized in the following format:

```
## 3.3.1.2 Compare run means and variances
## ydata is a dataframe in the following format:
## signal  donor_id  run_id ########
##    XX       1         1      ########
##    XX       1         2      ########
##    ...     ...       ...     ########
##    XX       1         J      ########
##    XX       2         1      ########
##    ...     ...       ...     ########
##    ...     ...       ...     ########
##    ...     ...       ...     ########
##    XX       I         J      ########
ydata$donor_id<-factor(ydata$donor_id)
ydata$run_id<-factor(ydata$run_id)
```

The *factor* function makes sure donor_id and run_id are treated as group labels, not numerical values.

To compare the equality of run means, the function *aov* is used for ANOVA analysis. The *aov* function essentially calls the linear regression function *lm*. To obtain estimate of run means, call the linear regression function *lm* by adding "-1" in the model specification to exclude the intercept. Note that by doing this, the resultant F-test from this linear regression fit has degree-of-freedom J instead of $J - 1$. F-test from *aov* output should be used to test the equality of run means.

```
anova.fit<-aov(signal~run_id,data=ydata)
lm.fit<-lm(signal~run_id-1,data=ydata)
summary(anova.fit)
summary(lm.fit)
```

Testing equality of run variances using Levene's test or Brown–Forsythe test can be achieved by utilizing function *levene.test* in the `lawstat` package. As shown below, when the location parameter is specified as "mean", the Levene's test is performed; when the location parameter is specified as "median", the actual test is Brown–Forsythe test.

```
## Test of variance equality
library(lawstat)
## Levene's test
levene.test(signal,run_id,location="mean",data=ydata)
## Brown-Forsythe test
levene.test(signal,run_id,location="median",data=ydata)
```

To estimate the mean and standard deviation of donor response from each run, simply use function *mean* and *sd*. The robust counterparts are *median* and *mad*. By default, the constant coefficient 1.483 has already been included in the output from *mad*. The cut point for each run can be calculated accordingly as in section 3.3.1.3. A mixed-effect ANOVA model (Equation (3.10)) can be fitted by calling the function *lme* in package `nlme`. The function *VarCorr* extracts all the variance components including that of the residuals.

```
library(nlme)
mixed.fit<-lme(fixed=signal~run_id,random=~1|donor_id)
     ## variance components
Var<-VarCorr(mixed.fit)
Var<-as.numeric(Var[,1])
```

In function *lme*, fixed effects and random effects are specified separately. The *lmer* function in package `lme4` can also be used to fit mixed-effect model, but the model specification grammar is different.

```
library(lme4)
mixed.fit2<-lmer(signal~run_id+(1|donor_id))
```

6.3 Implementation of Statistical Analysis of Clinical Immunogenicity Assessment

6.3.1 Statistical Analysis of ADA Status

The data set `ADASUMMARY` includes the following four variables

- `Recurrence` is the binary endpoint for RA recurrence

- `DoseGroup` is a categorical variable for dose level

- `ADAStatus` is a binary variable for binary ADA status

- `RecurrenceTime` is the time of recurrence of RA symptoms

The format of the variables are below:

```
proc format;
 value DoseGroupf
       0='Placebo'
       1='10 mg'
       2='20 mg'
       3='40 mg'
 ;
 value ADAfmt
       1='+'
       0='-'
 ;
run;
```

The confidence interval of the ADA response rates based on the logit scale can be calculated as

```
proc surveyfreq data=ADASUMMARY;
 table ADAStatus/cl (type=logit);
 by DoseGroup;
run;
```

To compare and test the difference of ADA response rates between different dose groups, one can use the `Proc Freq`. The option `all` in the `table` statement indicates all statistical tests of association will be calculated.

```
data TestADA;
input DoseGroup ADA Count;
cards;
0 0 142
```

```
0 1   8
1 0 125
1 1  25
2 0 110
2 1  40
3 0  90
3 1  60
;
run;

/* Statistical test between placebo and 10mg group */
proc freq data=TestADA;
 table DoseGroup*ADA/all;
 weight count;
 where DoseGroup in (0,1);
run;
```

6.3.2   Effects of ADA on Drug Efficacy

The following example illustrates the Cochran–Mantel–Haenszel (CMH) test to assess the effect of ADA on binary RA recurrence after stratifying by the dose level.

```
title 'Cochran-Mantel-Haenszel test';
proc freq data=ADASUMMARY;
 table DoseGroup*ADAStatus*Recurrence/cmh;
run;
```

The effect of ADA on censored survival outcomes can be tested using SAS Proc Lifetest or R function survfit(). The following code demonstrates the use of R function. We assume that in the data set, the right-censored time of RA recurrence is RecurrenceTime and the binary censored status is Recurrence. The Cox proportional-hazards model can be fitted using SAS Proc phreg or R function coxph().

```
# Fit the Kaplan-Meier survival curves by ADA status
Surv.by.ADA<-survfit(Surv(RecurrenceTime,Recurrence)~ADAStatus,
+ data=RAData)

# Plots of the survival curves
plot(Surv.by.ADA,ylim=c(0.6,1),ylab="% of staying remission",
+ xlab="Time (day)",lty=1:2,col=c("black","blue"))

# Log-rank test the difference of survival by ADA status,
# stratified by Dose Group
```

```
survdiff(Surv(RecurrenceTime,Recurrence)~ADAStatus+
+ strata(DoseGroup),data=RAData)

# cox proportional-hazards model
coxph(Surv(RecurrenceTime,Recurrence)~ADAStatus
+ *as.factor(DoseGroup),data=RAData)
```

For longitudinal data, the effects of drug and ADA response on longitudinal outcomes can be estimated using generalized estimating equations (GEE) or random-effects model. In the example, we assume that the variables in the longitudinal data set include

- `ADAStatus`: Overall binary variable for ADA Status, ADAStatus=1 for ADA+ subjects

- `ADA`: time-specific binary ADA status at each follow-up time

- `Time`: follow-up time in weeks

- `DAS28`: DAS28 score for disease activity

- `ADATiter`: Numeric value of ADA titer

- `CharADATiter`: Character value of ADA Titer

The sample data and R code of fitting longitudinal model are shown below:

```
#===============================================================
# Data frame: RALongitudinalData                               #
# Sample data excerpt                                          #
# ID DoseGroup ADAStatus Time  AS28 ADA ADATiter CharADATiter  #
# 1    0          1        0    6    0    0         <10         #
# 1    0          1        7    5    1    20        20          #
# 1    0          1       14    5    1    40        40          #
# ...                                                          #
#===============================================================


# Marginal model for longitudinal outcome (GEE)
library(geepack)
gee.das<-geeglm(DAS28 ~ as.factor(DoseGroup)+
+ ADAStatus+Time+Time*as.factor(DoseGroup),
+ data = RALongitduinalData id = ID, corstr = "exchangeable")

# Mixed-effects model for longitudinal outcomes
library(lme4)
library(lmerTest)
lme.das<-lmer(DAS28 ~ as.factor(DoseGroup)+ADAStatus+Time+
+ Time*as.factor(DoseGroup)+(1|ID), data=RALongitudinalData)
```

```
# Generalized additive models by dose group=i and ADA status=k
# i=0,1,2,3 and k=0,1
library(mgcv)
TDAS<-RALongitudinalData[RALongitudinalData$DoseGroup==i
+    & RALongitudinalData$ADAStatus==k,]
gamm.fit<-gamm(DAS28~ns(Time,df=2),random=list(ID=~1),
                 data=TDAS)
gamm.pred<-predict(gamm.fit$gam,type="response",se.fit=TRUE,
+    newdata=data.frame(Time=1:52))
```

6.3.3   Statistical Analysis of ADA Onset and Duration

Because of discrete observation of ADA status, the ADA onset time is interval-censored data. Let (LeftOnset,RightOnset] denote the intervals that the ADA onset times belong to. The four dose levels are dichotomized into two groups, e.g., Group 1 = (placebo, 10mg) and Group 2 = (20mg and 40 mg). The interval-censored survival data can be analyzed using R function ICsurv.

```
library(ICsurv)
ADADuration$Group<-0+(ADADuration$DoseGroup>1)
onset.fit<-icfit(Surv(LeftOnset,RightOnset,type=
+ "interval2")~Group, data=ADADuration)

par(mar=c(4,4,1,1))
plot(onset.fit,XLAB="ADA onset time (month)",YLAB=
+ "Probability of subjects with no detectable ADA",
LEGEND=FALSE)
legend(x=0,y=0.2,c("Dose<=10mg","Dose>10mg"),lty=1:2)
```

6.3.4   Statistical Analysis of ADA Titer

Like the ADA onset time, the ADA titer is also an interval-censored variable. To estimate the mean and confidence interval of the titer, one often assumes a log-normal distribution for the titer value. The estimates can be obtained using SAS Proc lifereg. Let (TiterLowerRange, TiterUpperRange) denote the lower and upper range of the titer value.

```
proc lifereg data=ADASUMMARY;
 class DoseGroup;
 model (TiterLowerRange,TiterUpperRange)=DoseGroup
 + /dist=lognormal ;
 lsmeans DoseGroup/cl;
 ods output LSMeans=LSM;
run;
```

```
data LSM;
 set LSM;
 Estimate=exp(Estimate);
 Lower=exp(Lower);
 Upper=exp(Upper);
 keep DoseGroup Estimate Lower Upper;
run;

title 'MLE of the mean and confidence interval of titer
+ based on the log-normal distribution';
proc print data=LSM;
 var DoseGroup Estimate Lower Upper;
 format DoseGroup dosegroupf. Estimate Lower Upper f7.0;
run;
```

6.4 Graphical Tools for Cause and Effect and Design Space Analysis

6.4.1 Ishikawa Diagram

The Ishikawa diagram also known as the fishbone diagram is an effective tool for visualizing the relationships between risk factors and immunogenicity responses. The diagram lists the inputs (causes) such as product-related parameters and the output (effects) such as ADA incidence rate. The function cause.and.effect in qcc package can be handily used to create the fishbone diagram. Figure 5.2.1 is generated using the following R code.

```
library(qcc)
cause.and.effect(cause=list(
"Product-related"=c("Molecular structure", "Glycosylation",
+ "Aggregates", "Oxidation","Deamination"),
"Process-related"=c("Impurities","Host-cell proteins",
+ "Host-cell DNA","Process change"),
"Patient-related"=c("Immunologic status","Prior sensitization",
+ "Age","Gender"),
"Treatment-related"=c("Route of administration","Dose",
+ "Frequency","Genetic status")),
"effect"="Immunogenicity Risk")
```

6.4.2   Pareto Plot

An equally commonly used graphical tool for cause and effect analysis is the Pareto plot. As previously described, the plot is based on the Pareto principle that states that among all the causes that may have effects on an outcome, roughly 20% of them cause 80% of the effects. The following shows how to use R function *pareto.chart* to create a Pareto plot.

```
risk.score =c(2,4,6,8,125,8,25,50,75,100,40,24,24,16)
names(risk.score) <-
c("Immunologic status", "Prior sensitization",
+ "Route of administration", "Genetic status",
+ "Endogenous protein", "Product origin",
+ "Post translation modification", "Aggregates",
+ "Glycosylation", "Impurity","Immunomodulation",
+ "Formulation", "Container closure", "Product custody")

pareto.chart(risk.score, main="Pareto Plot", ylab="Risk score",
+ col=heat.colors(length(risk.score)))

abline(h=(sum(risk.score)*.8),col="red",lwd=1)
```

6.4.3   Acceptance Region

In this section, we describe the use of function *wireframe* in R package `lattice` to depict the relationship between a risk response such as risk score and two critical quality attributes (CQAs). This serves as the foundation to devise a control strategy for the CQAs by defining a joint acceptance region. To this end, one needs to first establish a functional relationship between the risk response and the two CQAs. Let $p(x, y)$ denote such a function. An example is given in given in Section 5.3 where $p(x, y)$ is the risk score and x and y are median size and average content of residual DNA in the final dose of a drug, respectively. To plot $p(x, y)$ against (x, y), the response $p(x, y)$ is first evaluated over a grid of (x, y) coordinates, using the following R code.

```
x<-seq(1,1000,by=2)
y<-seq(1,100, by=2)
P<-matrix(0,nrow=length(x), ncol=length(y))
for(i in 1:length(x))
for(j in 1:length(y)) { P[i,j]=p(x[i], y[j])}
```

The R code listed below can then be used to create a three dimensional plot of $p(x, y)$ versus (x, y). However, both $p(x, y)$ and (x, y) coordinates created above need to be placed in vector forms before being used as inputs of function wireframe.

```
library(lattice)
t_x<-rep(x, length(y))
t_y<-rep(y, each=length(x))
wireframe(P~t_x*t_y, screen=list(z=-15,x=-65),drape=TRUE,
+ scales=list(arrows=FALSE,tck=0.5),
+ colorkey=FALSE,shade=TRUE,
+ xlab=list("CQA1",rot=-5,cex=0.8),
+ ylab=list("CQA2",rot=65,cex=0.8),
+ zlab=list("Risk response",rot=90))

library(lattice)
t_x<-rep(x, length(y))
t_y<-rep(y, each=length(x))
wireframe(P~t_x*t_y, screen=list(z=-15,x=-65), drape=TRUE,
+ scales=list(arrows=FALSE, tck=0.5),
+ colorkey=FALSE,shade=TRUE,
+ xlab=list("CQA1",rot=-5,cex=0.8),
+ ylab=list("CQA2",rot=65,cex=0.8),
+ zlab=list("Risk response",rot=90))
```

The acceptance region can be obtained in two steps: 1) Dichotomize the risk score P such that it is equal to zero if it is below a pre-specified acceptable limit; otherwise it is equal to one; 2) Plot the binary function, using R function *wireframe*. The acceptance range corresponds to combinations of (x, y) coordinates that produce $p(x, y)$ values equal to zero. Refer to Section 5.3 for a detailed application of this graphical tool.

6.5   Immunogenicity Biomarker Discovery

Immunogenicity biomarkers data can be nicely visualized using the *heatmap()* function as seen in Section 5.4. By default, the *heatmap()* function reorder the rows and columns of the biomarker data according to the row and column hierarchical clustering dendrogram. The color scheme can be passed to the function through the `col` parameter and advanced users can brew their own color schemes using the `RColorBrewer` package. The *heatmap.2()* function in the `gplots` package provides additional options to the standard *heatmap()* function. Since different biomarkers may have drastically different expression levels, they should be normalized before drawing the plot. This is easily done by using the option *scale="row"*. Assuming that each row of the biomarker data represents a biomarker and each column represents a sample, the following code generates a heatmap plot using classic red-green color scheme without showing the dendrogram.

```
heatmap.2(data, col=redgreen(75), scale="row",ColSideColors=cc,
+ labRow=NA,RowSideColors=rc,Rowv=NA,Colv=NA,dendrogram="none",
+ key=T,symkey=F,density.info="none",trace="none")
```

Hierarchical clustering method is an import tool to identify biomarker modules and sample groups. Correlation is preferably used as the distance measure between different biomarkers. Average linkage method is commonly used for defining the distance between modules.

```
diss=1-abs(cor(biomarker_data))
hier <- hclust(as.dist(diss),method="average")
```

The biomarker modules can be identified using the *cutree()* function supplied by R or by *cutTreeStatic()* function that can be downloaded from http://labs.genetics.ucla.edu/horvath/CoexpressionNetwork/MarcCarlson/NetworkFunctionsForYEAST.txt. The *cutTreeStatic()* function has many advantages over the generic *cutree()* function. It can detect modules not only by the hight in the dendrogram, but also it provides an option to refine modules based on their sizes.

The regression tree method can be readily deployed using *rpart()* function.

```
fit.tree = rpart(as.factor(y)~., method="class",x=T, data=raw,
+ control = rpart.control(cp = 0.05))
```

6.6 Report Automation

All the analyses in this book are carried out using either R or SAS code. In this section, we demonstrate useful techniques to automate statistical report. Routine analysis reports can be and should be automated. The purpose of an automated report system is to enable the scientist, who does the experiment and generate the data, to conduct a statistical analysis and write an analysis report. The automated system saves statisticians time and efforts to engage in those activities that should be handled best by the scientists themselves. On the other hand, the scientists welcome the automated system as well because they can get the report to them fast with only a mouse click. We have tested several report automation tools and only recently managed to generate reports with satisfactory quality. In our experience, the biggest difficulty to generate a high quality report is not producing the text, table, or the figure, it is however how to properly place those items in the right location of a file. Different R packages offer different levels of format control. In the following, we show how to generate a report in Pdf, rtf, and docx formats.

6.6.1 Generate Reports in pdf, rtf, and docx Formats

`knitr` is an R package that allows user to seamlessly write text and executable R code in one single Latex file. This file can then be compiled into a pdf file using *knit2pdf* command in R. The R code starts with <<>>= and end with @. For example, if the user wants to report the mean and variance of a random variable, he can write in an .Rnw file as

```
<<eval=TRUE, echo=FALSE>>=    ## start R code
set.seed(1)
x=rnorm(100)
mu=mean(x)
sigma2=var(x)
@                             ## end R code

The mean of X is \Sexpr{mu} and the variance of X is
\Sexpr{sigma2}.
```

After the the file is compiled to a pdf file, the output in the report looks like

The mean of X is -0.0378 and the variance of X is 0.9175.

The plot can be created on the fly as well. Following code gives a simple example of drawing a scatter plot.

```
<<fig.width=4, fig.height=4, out.width='.4\\linewidth',
+ echo=FALSE, results='asis'>>=
y=x+rnorm(100, 0, 0.5)
par(mar=c(4,4,.1,.1))
plot(x, y)
@
```

The result of an analysis can be nicely summarized using xtable() command as shown in the below example.

```
<<tidy=TRUE, echo=FALSE, results='asis'>>=
lm1=lm(y~x)
xtable(summary(lm1))
@
```

TABLE 6.1
Summary of linear regression model fitting: lm1

	Estimate	Std. Error	t value	Pr($>$|t|)
(Intercept)	-0.0188	0.0485	-0.39	0.6984
x	0.9995	0.0539	18.56	0.0000

LaTeX is a mature publication system that generates a pdf file with all the desired effects one can imagine. Since `knitr` package knits R code with LaTeX commands, it takes full advantage of the entire capacity that Latex can offer. The only issue with a pdf file is that it is difficult to edit after creation. `rtf` and `R2DOCX` are two alternative packages worth mentioning here. RTF stands for Rich Text Format, which gives users access to edit the file and convert the file to a pdf or a docx file. The rtf package in R has a set of commands that can add text, figure, table, and do limited format controls. These commands include

```
addHeader()
addParagraph()
addText()
addTable()
addPlot()
...
```

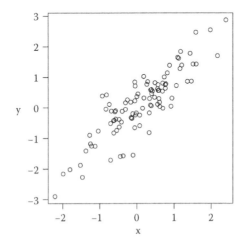

FIGURE 6.3
Simple scatter plot.

Although `rtf` package can create editable files, its format control functions are very limited and it is not flexible enough to generate a high quality document. However it is easy to use and is suitable to produce less format demanding documents. To generate documents with challenging formats, we found the `R2DOCX` package is perfect for the task. `R2DOCX` package offers two methods to output a MS Word docx file. The first method is to use functions to write items directly to the file. `R2DOCX` uses the same function names, *addParagraph()*, *addTable()*, *addPlot()*, as the `rtf` package to add text, table, and figure. However, these functions are more flexible. For example, the *addParagraph()* function not only provides options to output the text in different preset styles, it also provides options to change font size, color, and type of the whole or part of a sentence. The *addTable()* function gives the user full control of grouping columns, merging cells, and coloring cell background and font.

The second method offered by `R2DOCX` package is to allow users to replace bookmarks in a template file with text, table, or figure. In our opinion, this option makes the package superior to all other packages. For example, one can create a bookmarker, `BK1`, in a template file as a place holder, and then use *addParagraph(template, value=new_paragraph,stylename="Normal", bookmark="BK1")* function to replace the bookmark using the paragraph created in the R program. Since the bookmark can be placed in any places of the file, including the header, the footer,and any cell in a table, the template itself can be used to fix all formats that is necessary for the report. If special formatting issues remain to be addressed after the report being generated, one can easily use MS Word Macro to solve all of them in one sweep.

6.6.2   Shiny Server: Online Report Generation

Since most scientists do not have proper training for coding complicated analysis, it is no appropriate to release the code to them to do the analysis and generate the report. We find out that the Shiny Server is an ideal low cost solution for statistical analysis and report automation. Shiny Server is developed by Rstudio and the Open Source Edition is free of charge. The Professional Edition with 20 concurrent users is merely $9,995 a year, considerably cheaper than other softwares. The Shiny Server can be simply hosted in a Ubuntu desktop and the automation tools implemented on the Shiny Server can be accessed by the intended users through web browsers.

With the implementation of the web-based automation system, the statisticians can put more effort to improve the system to make it more user friendly. On the other hand, the scientists can get their reports whenever and wherever necessary. It is a truly win-win situation.

Bibliography

Adair, F. and D. Ozanne (2002). The immunogenicity of therapeutic proteins. *BioPharm 15*(2), 30–36.

Agarwal, S. K. (2011). Biologic agents in rheumatoid arthritis: An update for managed care professionals. *Journal of Managed Care Pharmacy 17*(9), S14.

Agoram, B. M. (2009). Use of pharmacokinetic/pharmacodynamic modelling for starting dose selection in first-in-human trials of high-risk biologics. *British Journal of Clinical Pharmacology 67*(2), 153–160.

Agresti, A. (2014). *Categorical Data Analysis*. Wiley Series in Probability and Statistics. John Wiley & Sons.

Al Arfaj, A. S., A. Rauf Chowdhary, N. Khalil, and R. Ali (2007). Immunogenicity of singlet oxygen modified human DNA: Implications for anti-DNA antibodies in systemic lupus erythematosus. *Clinical Immunology 124*(1), 83–89.

Andersen, P. K., J. P. Klein, K. M. Knudsen, and R. T. y Palacios (1997). Estimation of variance in Cox's regression model with shared gamma frailties. *Biometrics*, 1475–1484.

Andreev, A. and E. Arjas (1998). Acute middle ear infection in small children: A Bayesian analysis using multiple time scales. *Lifetime Data Analysis 4*(2), 121–137.

Armitage, P. (1955). Tests for linear trends in proportions and frequencies. *Biometrics 11*(3), 375–386.

Atkinson, G. and A. Nevill (1997). Comment on the use of concordance correlation to assess the agreement between two variables. *Biometrics 53*(2), 775–777.

Azzalini, A. and A. Capitanio (2003). Distributions generated by perturbation of symmetry with emphasis on a multivariate skew *t*-distribution. *Journal of the Royal Statistical Society: Series B (Statistical Methodology) 65*(2), 367–389.

Bacchetti, P. (1990). Estimating the incubation period of AIDS by comparing population infection and diagnosis patterns. *Journal of the American Statistical Association 85*, 1002–1008.

Baker, M., H. Reynolds, B. Lumicisi, and C. Bryson (2010). Immunogenicity of protein therapeutics: The key causes, consequences and challenges. *Self Nonself 1*(4), 314–322.

Barbosa, M. D., C. R. Gleason, K. R. Phillips, F. Berisha, B. Stouffer, B. M. Warrack, and G. Chen (2012). Addressing drug effects on cut point determination for an anti-drug antibody assay. *Journal of Immunological Methods 384*(1), 152–156.

Barnhart, H. X., A. S. Kosinski, and M. J. Haber (2007). Assessing individual agreement. *Journal of Biopharmaceutical Statistics 17*(4), 697–719.

Bastian, D., H. Borel, T. Sasaki, A. Steinberg, and Y. Borel (1985). Immune response to nucleic acid antigens and native DNA by human peripheral blood lymphocytes *in vitro*. *The Journal of Immunology 135*(3), 1772–1777.

Benjamini, Y. and Y. Hochberg (1995). Controlling the false discovery rate: A practical and powerful approach to multiple testing. *Journal of the Royal Statistical Society. Series B (Statistical Methodology)*, 289–300.

Berger, R. L. and J. C. Hsu (1996). Bioequivalence trials, intersection-union tests and equivalence confidence sets. *Statistical Science 11*(4), 283–319.

Berry, S. M. and D. A. Berry (2004). Accounting for multiplicities in assessing drug safety: A three-level hierarchical mixture model. *Biometrics 60*(2), 418–426.

Bland, J. and D. Altman (1986). Statistical methods for assessing agreement between two methods of clinical measurement. *The Lancet 327*(8476), 307–310.

Bland, J. M. and D. G. Altman (1999). Measuring agreement in method comparison studies. *Statistical Methods in Medical Research 8*(2), 135–160.

Bonate, P. L., C. Sung, K. Welch, and S. Richards (2009). Conditional modeling of antibody titers using a zero-inflated poisson random effects model: Application to Fabrazyme®. *Journal of Pharmacokinetics and Pharmacodynamics 36*(5), 443–459.

Bonett, D. G. (2002). Sample size requirements for estimating intraclass correlations with desired precision. *Statistics in Medicine 21*(9), 1331–1335.

Booth, J. G. and J. P. Hobert (1999). Maximizing generalized linear mixed model likelihoods with an automated Monte Carlo EM algorithm. *Journal of the Royal Statistical Society: Series B (Statistical Methodology) 61*(1), 265–285.

Borgan, Ø. (2005). Nelson–Aalen estimator. *Encyclopedia of Biostatistics*.

Bossaller, L. and A. Rothe (2013). Monoclonal antibody treatments for rheumatoid arthritis. *Expert Opinion on Biological Therapy 13*(9), 1257–1272.

Box, G. E. and D. W. Behnken (1960). Some new three level designs for the study of quantitative variables. *Technometrics 2*(4), 455–475.

Box, G. E. and D. R. Cox (1964). An analysis of transformations. *Journal of the Royal Statistical Society. Series B (Methodological)*, 211–252.

Box, G. E., J. S. Hunter, and W. G. Hunter (2005). *Statistics for Experimenters: Design, Innovation, and Discovery*. Wiley-Interscience; 2nd edition.

Breslow, N. (1974). Covariance analysis of censored survival data. *Biometrics*, 89–99.

Breslow, N. E. and D. G. Clayton (1993). Approximate inference in generalized linear mixed models. *Journal of the American Statistical Association 88*(421), 9–25.

Breslow, N. E. and N. E. Day (1987). *Statistical Methods in Cancer Research*, Volume 2. International Agency for Research on Cancer, Lyon.

Brinks, V., W. Jiskoot, and H. Schellekens (2011). Immunogenicity of therapeutic proteins: The use of animal models. *Pharmaceutical Research 28*(10), 2379–2385.

Brown, E. G., L. Wood, and S. Wood (1999). The medical dictionary for regulatory activities (MedDRA). *Drug Safety 20*(2), 109–117.

Brown, M. B. and A. B. Forsythe (1974). Robust tests for the equality of variances. *Journal of the American Statistical Association 69*(346), 364–367.

Brusic, V., G. Rudy, G. Honeyman, J. Hammer, and L. Harrison (1998). Prediction of MHC class ii-binding peptides using an evolutionary algorithm and artificial neural network. *Bioinformatics 14*(2), 121–130.

Bunkley, N. (March 3, 2008). Joseph Juran, 103, pioneer in quality control, dies. *New York Times*.

Cao, D. and X. He (2011). Statistical analysis of adverse events in randomized clinical trials using SAS. *PharmaSUG* (SP07).

Casadevall, N., J. Nataf, B. Viron, A. Kolta, J.-J. Kiladjian, P. Martin-Dupont, P. Michaud, T. Papo, V. Ugo, I. Teyssandier, et al. (2002). Pure red-cell aplasia and antierythropoietin antibodies in patients treated with recombinant erythropoietin. *New England Journal of Medicine 346*(7), 469–475.

Chamberlain, P. (2008). Presenting an immunogenicity risk assessment to regulatory agencies. In *Immunogenicity of Biopharmaceuticals*, pp. 239–258. Springer.

Chamberlain, P. (2011, Jan). Addressing immunogenicity-related risks in an integrated manner. Dossier Strategy.

Chen, D. and K. Peace (2013). *Applied Meta-Analysis with R*. Chapman & Hall/CRC Biostatistics Series. Taylor & Francis.

Chen, D.-G. D., J. Sun, and K. E. Peace (2012). *Interval-Censored Time-to-Event Data: Methods and Applications*. CRC Press.

Chen, K. and M. Zhou (2003). Non-parametric hypothesis testing and confidence intervals with doubly censored data. *Lifetime Data Analysis 9*(1), 71–91.

Chen, X. C., L. Zhou, S. Gupta, and F. Civoli (2012). Implementation of design of experiments (DOE) in the development and validation of a cell-based bioassay for the detection of anti-drug neutralizing antibodies in human serum. *Journal of Immunological Methods 376*(1), 32–45.

Chow, S.-C. (2013). *Biosimilars: Design and Analysis of Follow-on Biologics*. CRC Press.

Chuang-Stein, C. (1998). Safety analysis in controlled clinical trials. *Drug Information Journal 32*(1 suppl), 1363S–1372S.

Chuang-Stein, C., V. Le, and W. Chen (2001). Recent advancements in the analysis and presentation of safety data. *Drug Information Journal 35*(2), 377–397.

Chuang-Stein, C. and N. Mohberg (1993). A unified approach to analyze safety data in clinical trials. *Drug Safety Assessment in Clinical Trials*.

Civoli, F., M. A. Kroenke, K. Reynhardt, Y. Zhuang, A. Kaliyaperumal, and S. Gupta (2012). Development and optimization of neutralizing antibody assays to monitor clinical immunogenicity. *Bioanalysis 4*(22), 2725–2735.

Clayton, D. G. (1978). A model for association in bivariate life tables and its application in epidemiological studies of familial tendency in chronic disease incidence. *Biometrika 65*(1), 141–151.

CMC Biotech Working Group (2009). A-mab: A case study in bioprocess development.

CMC Vaccine Working Group (2012). A-vax: Applying quality by design to vaccines.

Cochran, W. G. (1954a). The combination of estimates from different experiments. *Biometrics 10*(1), 101–129.

Cochran, W. G. (1954b). Some methods for strengthening the common χ^2 tests. *Biometrics 10*(4), 417–451.

Cornips, C. and H. Schellekens (2010). Biomarkers for the immunogenicity of therapeutic proteins and its clinical consequences. *Pharmaceutical Sciences Encyclopedia*.

Cox, D. and D. Oakes (1984). *Analysis of Survival Data.* Chapman & Hall/CRC Monographs on Statistics & Applied Probability. Taylor & Francis.

Cox, D. R. (1972). Regression Models and Life-Tables. *Journal of the Royal Statistical Society. Series B (Methodological) 34*(2), 187–220.

Cross, M., E. Smith, D. Hoy, L. Carmona, F. Wolfe, T. Vos, B. Williams, S. Gabriel, M. Lassere, N. Johns, et al. (2014). The global burden of rheumatoid arthritis: estimates from the global burden of disease 2010 study. *Annals of the Rheumatic Diseases 73*(7), 1316–1322.

Davidian, M. and D. Giltinan (1995). *Nonlinear Models for Repeated Measurement Data.* Chapman & Hall/CRC Monographs on Statistics & Applied Probability. Taylor & Francis.

De Groot, A. S. and W. Martin (2009). Reducing risk, improving outcomes: bioengineering less immunogenic protein therapeutics. *Clinical Immunology 131*(2), 189–201.

De Gruttola, V. and S. W. Lagakos (1989). Analysis of doubly-censored survival data, with application to AIDS. *Biometrics*, 1–11.

Dempster, A. P., N. M. Laird, and D. B. Rubin (1977). Maximum likelihood from incomplete data via the em algorithm. *Journal of the Royal Statistical Society. Series B (Methodological)*, 1–38.

DerSimonian, R. and R. Kacker (2007). Random-effects model for meta-analysis of clinical trials: An update. *Contemporary Clinical Trials 28*(2), 105–114.

DerSimonian, R. and N. Laird (1986). Meta-analysis in clinical trials. *Controlled Clinical Trials 7*(3), 177–188.

Devanarayan, V. and M. G. Tovey (2011). Cut points and performance characteristics for anti-drug antibody assays. *Detection and Quantification of Antibodies to Biopharmaceuticals: Practical and Applied Considerations*, 287–308.

Dobson, A. and A. Barnett (2008). *An Introduction to Generalized Linear Models, Third Edition*. Chapman & Hall/CRC Texts in Statistical Science. Taylor & Francis.

Dodge, R., C. Daus, and D. Yaskanin (2009). Challenges in developing antidrug antibody screening assays. *Bioanalysis 1*(4), 699–704.

Dudoit, S., J. Fridlyand, and T. P. Speed (2002). Comparison of discrimination methods for the classification of tumors using gene expression data. *Journal of the American Statistical Association 97*(457), 77–87.

DuMouchel, W. (2012). Multivariate Bayesian logistic regression for analysis of clinical study safety issues. *Statistical Science 27*(3), 319–339.

Durrett, R. (2010). *Probability: Theory and Examples*. Cambridge Series in Statistical and Probabilistic Mathematics. Cambridge University Press.

EMA (2006, March). Guideline on clinical investigation of medicinal products other than NSAIDs for treatment. European Medicines Agency (EMA), committee for medicinal products for human use (CHMP).

EMA (2007). Guideline on immunogenicity assessment of biotechnology-derived therapeutic proteins. *London: European Medicines Agency*.

EMA (2012). Guideline on similar biological medicinal products containing monoclonal antibodies–non-clinical and clinical issues. *London: European Medicines Agency*.

EMA (2013). Guideline on similar biological medicinal products. *London: European Medicines Agency*.

EMA (2014, February). Concept paper on the revision of the guideline on immunogenicity assessment of biotechnology-derived therapeutic proteins (chmp/bmwp/42832/2005). Draft EMA/275542/2013, European Medicines Agency.

Fan, P. and K. Leong (2007). The use of biological agents in the treatment of rheumatoid arthritis. *Annals of the Academy of Medicine, Singapore 36*(2), 128.

Fay, M. P. (1996). Rank invariant tests for interval censored data under the grouped continuous model. *Biometrics*, 811–822.

Fay, M. P. and P. A. Shaw (2010). Exact and asymptotic weighted logrank tests for interval censored data: The `interval` R package. *Journal of Statistical Software 36*(2), 1–34.

FDA (1996). Guidance for industry: E6 good clinical practice: consolidated guidance. *Food and Drug Administration*.

FDA (2001). Guidance for industry: Statistical approaches to establishing bioequivalence. *Rockville, MD: U.S. Food and Drug Administration.*

FDA (2009). Guidance for industry: Assay development for immunogenicity testing of therapeutic proteins. *Food and Drug Administration.*

FDA (2013). Draft guidance for industry: Bioanalytical method validation. *Food and Drug Administration.*

FDA (2014). Guidance for industry: Immunogenicity assessment for therapeutic protein products. *USA: FDA Guidance Document.*

Felson, D. T., J. J. Anderson, M. L. Lange, G. Wells, and M. P. LaValley (1998). Should imporvement in rheumatoid arthritis clinical trials be defined as fifty percent or seventy percent improvement in core set measures, rather than twenty percent? *Arthritis & Rheumatism 41*(9), 1564–1570.

Findlay, J. W. and R. F. Dillard (2007). Appropriate calibration curve fitting in ligand binding assays. *The AAPS Journal 9*(2), E260–E267.

Finkelstein, D. M. (1986). A proportional hazards model for interval-censored failure time data. *Biometrics*, 845–854.

Fisher, R. A. (1922). On the interpretation of $\chi2$ from contingency tables, and the calculation of p. *Journal of the Royal Statistical Society*, 87–94.

Fleiss, J. L. and J. A. Berlin (2009). Effect sizes for dichotomous data.

Fleming, T. and D. Harrington (2011). *Counting Processes and Survival Analysis.* Wiley Series in Probability and Statistics. John Wiley & Sons.

Foged, C. and A. Sundblad (2008). Immune reactions towards biopharmaceuticals–a general, mechanistic overview. In *Immunogenicity of Biopharmaceuticals*, pp. 1–25. Springer.

Frydman, H. (1992). A nonparametric estimation procedure for a periodically observed three-state markov process, with application to AIDS. *Journal of the Royal Statistical Society, Series B 54*, 853–866.

Frydman, H. (1995). Semiparametric estimation in a three-state duration-dependent markov model from interval-censored observations with application to AIDS data. *Biometrics 51*(2), 502–511.

Garcês, S., J. Demengeot, and E. Benito-Garcia (2013). The immunogenicity of anti-tnf therapy in immune-mediated inflammatory diseases: A systematic review of the literature with a meta-analysis. *Annals of the Rheumatic Diseases 72*(12), 1947–1955.

Garsd, A., G. E. Ford, G. O. W. 3rd., and L. S. Rosenblatt (1983). Sample size for estimating the quantiles of endothelial cell-area distribution. *Biometrics 39*(2), 385–394.

Geng, D., G. Shankar, A. Schantz, M. Rajadhyaksha, H. Davis, and C. Wagner (2005). Validation of immunoassays used to assess immunogenicity to therapeutic monoclonal antibodies. *Journal of Pharmaceutical and Biomedical Analysis 39*(3), 364–375.

Gentleman, R. and C. J. Geyer (1994). Maximum likelihood for interval censored data: Consistency and computation. *Biometrika 81*(3), 618–623.

Gilkeson, G. S., J. P. Grudier, D. G. Karounos, and D. S. Pisetsky (1989). Induction of anti-double stranded DNA antibodies in normal mice by immunization with bacterial DNA. *The Journal of Immunology 142*(5), 1482–1486.

Gill, R. (1980). Censoring and stochastic integrals. *Statistica Neerlandica 34*(2), 124–124.

Glass, G. V. (1976). Primary, secondary, and meta-analysis of research. *Educational researcher*, 3–8.

Goetghebeur, E. and L. Ryan (2000). Semiparametric regression analysis of interval-censored data. *Biometrics 56*(4), 1139–1144.

Goggins, W. B., D. M. Finkelstein, D. A. Schoenfeld, and A. M. Zaslavsky (1998). A Markov chain Monte Carlo EM algorithm for analyzing interval-censored data under the Cox proportional hazards model. *Biometrics*, 1498–1507.

Goggins, W. B., D. M. Finkelstein, and A. M. Zaslavsky (1999). Applying the cox proportional hazards model for analysis of latency data with interval censoring. *Statistics in Medicine 18*(20), 2737–2747.

Gomez, G. and S. W. Lagakos (1994). Estimation of the infection time and latency distribution of AIDS with doubly censored data. *Biometrics 50*(1), 204–212.

Gorovits, B. (2009). Antidrug antibody assay validation: Industry survey results. *The AAPS Journal 11*(1), 133–138.

Groeneboom, P., M. H. Maathuis, and J. A. Wellner (2008). Current status data with competing risks: Consistency and rates of convergence of the mle. *The Annals of Statistics*, 1031–1063.

Guilford-Blake, R. and D. Strickland (2008). Guide to biotechnology. *Biotechnology Industry Organization*, 38.

Gupta, S., V. Devanarayan, D. Finco, G. R. Gunn III, S. Kirshner, S. Richards, B. Rup, A. Song, and M. Subramanyam (2011). Recommendations for the validation of cell-based assays used for the detection of neutralizing antibody immune responses elicited against biological therapeutics. *Journal of Pharmaceutical and Biomedical Analysis 55*(5), 878–888.

Gupta, S., S. R. Indelicato, V. Jethwa, T. Kawabata, M. Kelley, A. R. Mire-Sluis, S. M. Richards, B. Rup, E. Shores, and S. J. Swanson (2007). Recommendations for the design, optimization, and qualification of cell-based assays used for the detection of neutralizing antibody responses elicited to biological therapeutics. *Journal of Immunological Methods 321*(1), 1–18.

Haaland, P. D. (1989). *Experimental Design in Biotechnology*, Volume 105. CRC press.

Haight, F. A. and F. A. Haight (1967). *Handbook of the Poisson Distribution*. Wiley New York.

Halekoh, U., S. Højsgaard, and J. Yan (2006). The R package geepack for generalized estimating equations. *Journal of Statistical Software 15*(2), 1–11.

Hastie, T. J. and R. J. Tibshirani (1990). *Generalized Additive Models*, Volume 43. CRC Press.

Hayakawa, T. and A. Ishii-Watabe (2011). Japanese regulatory perspective on immunogenicity. *Detection and Quantification of Antibodies to Biopharmaceuticals: Practical and Applied Considerations*, 57–79.

Hedges, L. V. and J. L. Vevea (1998). Fixed-and random-effects models in meta-analysis. *Psychological Methods 3*(4), 486.

Heidelberger, P. and P. D. Welch (1983). Simulation run length control in the presence of an initial transient. *Operations Research 31*(6), 1109–1144.

Henschel, V., C. Heiß, and U. Mansmann (2009). intcox: Compendium to apply the iterative convex minorant algorithm to interval censored event data.

Hider, S. L., C. Buckley, A. J. Silman, D. Symmons, and I. N. Bruce (2005). Factors influencing response to disease modifying antirheumatic drugs in patients with rheumatoid arthritis. *Journal of Rheumatology 32*(1), 11–16.

Hoffman, D. (2010). One-sided tolerance limits for balanced and unbalanced random effects models. *Technometrics 52*(3).

Hoffman, D. and M. Berger (2011). Statistical considerations for calculation of immunogenicity screening assay cut points. *Journal of Immunological Methods 373*(1), 200–208.

Hoffmann, S., S. Cepok, V. Grummel, K. Lehmann-Horn, J. Hackermueller, P. F. Stadler, H.-P. Hartung, A. Berthele, F. Deisenhammer, R. Wasmuth, et al. (2008). Hla-drb1 *0401 and hla-drb1 0408 are strongly associated with the development of antibodies against interferon-β therapy in multiple sclerosis. *The American Journal of Human Genetics 83*(2), 219–227.

Hollander, M. and D. Wolfe (1999). *Nonparametric Statistical Methods*. Wiley Series in Probability and Statistics. John Wiley & Sons.

Horne, A. D. (1995). The statistical analysis of immunognicity data in vaccine atials. *Annals of the New York Academy of Sciences 754*(1), 329–346.

Hougaard, P. (1986). Survival models for heterogeneous populations derived from stable distributions. *Biometrika 73*(2), 387–396.

Huang, J. and J. A. Wellner (1997). Interval censored survival data: A review of recent progress. *Proceedings of the First Seattle Symposium in Biostatistics: Survival Analysis*, 123–169.

Hutson, A. D. (2003). Nonparametric estimation of normal ranges given one-way anova random effects assumptions. *Statistics & Probability Letters 64*(4), 415–424.

Hwang, W. Y. K. and J. Foote (2005). Immunogenicity of engineered antibodies. *Methods 36*(1), 3–10.

Ibrahim, J., M. Chen, and D. Sinha (2001). *Bayesian Survival Analysis*. Springer.

ICH (2005). Quality risk management Q9. *ICH Harmonized Tripartite Guideline, ICH Steering Committee.*

ICH (2008). Pharmaceutical quality system Q10. *ICH Harmonized Tripartite Guideline,ICH Steering Committee.*

ICH (2009). Pharmaceutical development Q8 (R2). *ICH Harmonized Tripartite Guideline, ICH Steering Committee 4.*

ICH (2011). Preclinical safety evaluation of biotechnology-derived pharmaceuticals S6 (R1),current step 4 version. *International Conference on Harmonization.*

Ishikawa, K. (1982). *Guide to Quality Control*, Volume 2. Asian Productivity Organization, Tokyo.

Jackson, D., J. Bowden, and R. Baker (2010). How does the DerSimonian and Laird procedure for random effects meta-analysis compare with its more efficient but harder to compute counterparts? *Journal of Statistical Planning and Inference 140*(4), 961–970.

Jaki, T., J.-P. Lawo, M. J. Wolfsegger, P. Allacher, and F. Horling (2014). A comparison of methods for classifying samples as truly specific with confirmatory immunoassays. *Journal of Pharmaceutical and Biomedical Analysis 88*, 27–35.

Jaki, T., J.-P. Lawo, M. J. Wolfsegger, J. Singer, P. Allacher, and F. Horling (2011). A formal comparison of different methods for establishing cut points to distinguish positive and negative samples in immunoassays. *Journal of Pharmaceutical and Biomedical Analysis 55*(5), 1148–1156.

Jara, A., F. Quintana, and E. San Martín (2008). Linear mixed models with skew-elliptical distributions: A Bayesian approach. *Computational Statistics & Data Analysis 52*(11), 5033–5045.

Jewell, N. P. (1994). Non-parametric estimation and doubly-censored data: General ideas and applications to AIDS. *Statistics in Medicine 13*(19-20), 2081–2095.

Jewell, N. P., H. M. Malani, and E. Vittinghoff (1994). Nonparametric estimation for a form of doubly censored data, with application to two problems in AIDS. *Journal of the American Statistical Association 89*, 7–18.

Joelsson, D., P. Moravec, M. Troutman, J. Pigeon, and P. DePhillips (2008). Optimizing ELISAs for precision and robustness using laboratory automation and statistical design of experiments. *Journal of Immunological Methods 337*(1), 35–41.

Johnson, N., S. Kotz, and N. Balakrishnan (1994). *Continuous Univariate Distributions, volume 1*. John Wiley & Sons.

Johnson, N., S. Kotz, and N. Balakrishnan (1995). *Continuous Univariate Distributions, volume 2*. John Wiley & Sons.

Jung, S.-H. (2014). Stratified Fisher's exact test and its sample size calculation. *Biometrical Journal 56*(1), 129–140.

Kalbfleisch, J. and R. Prentice (2002). *The Statistical Analysis of Failure Time Data*. Wiley Series in Probability and Statistics. John Wiley & Sons.

Kaplan, E. L. and P. Meier (1958). Nonparametric estimation from incomplete observations. *Journal of the American Statistical Association 53*(282), 457–481.

Karounos, D., J. Grudier, and D. Pisetsky (1988). Spontaneous expression of antibodies to dna of various species origin in sera of normal subjects and patients with systemic lupus erythematosus. *The Journal of Immunology 140*(2), 451–455.

Keiding, N. (2005). Delayed entry. *Encyclopedia of Biostatistics, 2nd Edition*.

Kirshner, S. (2011). Immunogenicity of therapeutic proteins: A regulatory perspective. *Detection and Quantification of Antibodies to Biopharmaceuticals: Practical and Applied Considerations*, 13–35.

Klein, J. and M. Moeschberger (2003). *Survival Analysis: Techniques for Censored and Truncated Data*. Statistics for Biology and Health. Springer.

Klinman, D. M., G. Yamshchikov, and Y. Ishigatsubo (1997). Contribution of CpG motifs to the immunogenicity of DNA vaccines. *The Journal of Immunology 158*(8), 3635–3639.

Kojima, Y., K.-Q. Xin, T. Ooki, K. Hamajima, T. Oikawa, K. Shinoda, T. Ozaki, Y. Hoshino, N. Jounai, M. Nakazawa, et al. (2002). Adjuvant effect of multi-CpG motifs on an HIV-1 DNA vaccine. *Vaccine 20*(23), 2857–2865.

Koren, E., H. W. Smith, E. Shores, G. Shankar, D. Finco-Kent, B. Rup, Y.-C. Barrett, V. Devanarayan, B. Gorovits, and S. Gupta (2008). Recommendations on risk-based strategies for detection and characterization of antibodies against biotechnology products. *Journal of Immunological Methods 333*(1), 1–9.

Krishnamoorthy, K. and T. Mathew (2009). *Statistical Tolerance Regions: Theory, Applications, and Computation*. John Wiley & Sons.

Kromminga, A. and G. Deray (2008). Case study: Immunogenicity of rhepo. In *Immunogenicity of Biopharmaceuticals*, pp. 113–126. Springer.

Kubiak, R. J., L. Zhang, J. Zhang, Y. Zhu, N. Lee, F. F. Weichold, H. Yang, V. Abraham, P. F. Akufongwe, and L. Hewitt (2013). Correlation of screening and confirmatory results in tiered immunogenicity testing by solution-phase bridging assays. *Journal of Pharmaceutical and Biomedical Analysis 74*, 235–245.

Kuus-Reichel, K., L. Grauer, L. Karavodin, C. Knott, M. Krusemeier, and N. Kay (1994). Will immunogenicity limit the use, efficacy, and future development of therapeutic monoclonal antibodies? *Clinical and Diagnostic Laboratory Immunology 1*(4), 365–372.

Lachin, J. (2014). *Biostatistical Methods: The Assessment of Relative Risks*. Wiley Series in Probability and Statistics. John Wiley & Sons.

Landis, J. R. and G. G. Koch (1977). The measurement of observer agreement for categorical data. *Biometrics*, 159–174.

Lawless, J. (1982). *Statistical Models and Methods for Lifetime Data*. John Wiley & Sons.

Lawless, J. F. (1980). Inference in the generalized gamma and log gamma distributions. *Technometrics 22*(3), 409–419.

Lee, J. W., W. C. Smith, G. D. Nordblom, and R. R. Bowsher (2003). Validation of assays for the bioanalysis of novel biomarkers: Practical recommendations for clinical investigation of new drug entities. *Drugs and the Pharmaceutical Sciences 132*, 119–148.

Levene, H. (1960). Robust tests for equality of variances. *Contributions to Probability and Statistics: Essays in Honor of Harold Hotelling 2*, 278–292.

Liang, K.-Y. and S. L. Zeger (1986). Longitudinal data analysis using generalized linear models. *Biometrika 73*(1), 13–22.

Lievre, M., M. Cucherat, and A. Leizorovicz (2002). Pooling, meta-analysis, and the evaluation of drug safety. *Trials 3*(1), 6.

Lin, L. I. (1989). A concordance correlation coefficient to evaluate reproducibility. *Biometrics*, 255–268.

Lin, L. I. (1992). Assay validation using the concordance correlation coefficient. *Biometrics*, 599–604.

Lin, L. I. (2000). Total deviation index for measuring individual agreement with applications in laboratory performance and bioequivalence. *Statistics in Medicine 19*(2), 255–270.

MacQueen, J. (1967). Some methods for classification and analysis of multivariate observations. In *Proceedings of the Fifth Berkeley Symposium on Mathematical Statistics and Probability*, Volume 1, pp. 281–297. California, USA.

Makinen, H., P. Hannonen, T. Sokka, et al. (2006). Definitions of remission for rheumatoid arthritis and review of selected clinical cohorts and randomised clinical trials for the rate of remission. *Clinical and Experimental Rheumatology 24*(6), S22.

Mäkinen, H., H. Kautiainen, P. Hannonen, and T. Sokka (2005). Is DAS28 an appropriate tool to assess remission in rheumatoid arthritis? *Annals of the Rheumatic Diseases 64*(10), 1410–1413.

Maneiro, J. R., E. Salgado, and J. J. Gomez-Reino (2013). Immunogenicity of monoclonal antibodies against tumor necrosis factor used in chronic immune-mediated inflammatory conditions: systematic review and meta-analysis. *JAMA Internal Medicine 173*(15), 1416–1428.

Mantel, N. and W. Haenszel (1959). Statistical aspects of the analysis of data from retrospective studies of disease. *Journal of the National Cancer Institute 22*(4), 719–748.

Marubini, E. and M. Valsecchi (2004). *Analysing Survival Data from Clinical Trials and Observational Studies*. Statistics in Practice. John Wiley & Sons.

McCullagh, P. and J. Nelder (1989). *Generalized Linear Models*. Monographs on statistics and applied probability. Chapman & Hall.

McCulloch, C. and S. Searle (2004). *Generalized, Linear, and Mixed Models*. John Wiley & Sons.

McCulloch, C. E. and J. M. Neuhaus (2011). Misspecifying the shape of a random effects distribution: Why getting it wrong may not matter. *Statistical Science 26*(3), 388–402.

McGilchrist, C. and C. Aisbett (1991). Regression with frailty in survival analysis. *Biometrics*, 461–466.

McMahan, C. and L. Wang (2014). A statistical package for regression analysis of interval-censored data under the semiparametric proportional hazards (ph) model.

Mehrotra, D. V. and A. J. Adewale (2012). Flagging clinical adverse experiences: Reducing false discoveries without materially compromising power for detecting true signals. *Statistics in Medicine 31*(18), 1918–1930.

Mehrotra, D. V. and J. F. Heyse (2004). Use of the false discovery rate for evaluating clinical safety data. *Statistical Methods in Medical Research 13*(3), 227–238.

Mire-Sluis, A. R., Y. C. Barrett, V. Devanarayan, E. Koren, H. Liu, M. Maia, T. Parish, G. Scott, G. Shankar, and E. Shores (2004). Recommendations for the design and optimization of immunoassays used in the detection of host antibodies against biotechnology products. *Journal of Immunological Methods 289*(1), 1–16.

Montgomery, D. C. (2008). *Design and Analysis of Experiments*. John Wiley & Sons.

Moulton, L. H. and N. A. Halsey (1995). A mixture model with detection limits for regression analyses of antibody response to vaccine. *Biometrics*, 1570–1578.

Myers, R. H., D. C. Montgomery, and C. M. Anderson-Cook (2009). *Response Surface Methodology: Process and Product Optimization Using Designed Experiments*. John Wiley & Sons.

Nauta, J. (2010). *Statistics in Clinical Vaccine Trials*. Springer.

Nauta, J. J. (2006). Eliminating bias in the estimation of the geometric mean of hi titres. *Biologicals 34*(3), 183–186.

Nauta, J. J. and I. A. de Bruijn (2006). On the bias in hi titers and how to reduce it. *Vaccine 24*(44), 6645–6646.

Neyer, L., J. Hiller, K. Gish, S. Keller, and I. Caras (2006). Confirming human antibody responses to a therapeutic monoclonal antibody using a statistical approach. *Journal of Immunological Methods 315*(1), 80–87.

Nielsen, M., C. Lundegaard, P. Worning, C. S. Hvid, K. Lamberth, S. Buus, S. Brunak, and O. Lund (2004). Improved prediction of MHC class I and class II epitopes using a novel Gibbs sampling approach. *Bioinformatics 20*(9), 1388–1397.

O'Connell, M., B. Belanger, and P. Haaland (1993). Calibration and assay development using the four-parameter logistic model. *Chemometrics and Intelligent Laboratory Systems 20*(2), 97–114.

O'Neill, R. T. (1995). Statistical concepts in the planning and evaluation of drug safety from clinical trials in drug development: Issues of international harmonization. *Statistics in Medicine 14*(9), 1117–1127.

Pan, W. (2001). A multiple imputation approach to regression analysis for doubly censored data with application to AIDS studies. *Biometrics 57*(4), 1245–1250.

Parish, T. H., D. Finco, and V. Devanarayan (2009). Development and validation of immunogenicity assays for preclinical and clinical studies. In M. N. Khan and J. W. Findlay (Eds.), *Ligand-Binding Assays*. John Wiley & Sons, Inc.

Peterson, J. J. (2008). A Bayesian approach to the ICH Q8 definition of design space. *Journal of Biopharmaceutical Statistics 18*(5), 959–975.

Peto, R. (1973). Experimental survival curves for interval-censored data. *Applied Statistics*, 86–91.

PhRMA (2013). Medicines in Development: Biologics.

Pinheiro, J. C. and E. C. Chao (2006). Efficient Laplacian and adaptive Gaussian quadrature algorithms for multilevel generalized linear mixed models. *Journal of Computational and Graphical Statistics 15*(1).

Pisetsky, D. S. (1997). Specificity and immunochemical properties of antibodies to bacterial DNA. *Methods: A Companion to Methods in Enzymology 11*(1), 55–61.

Ponce, R., L. Abad, L. Amaravadi, T. Gelzleichter, E. Gore, J. Green, S. Gupta, D. Herzyk, C. Hurst, I. A. Ivens, et al. (2009). Immunogenicity of biologically-derived therapeutics: assessment and interpretation of nonclinical safety studies. *Regulatory Toxicology and Pharmacology 54*(2), 164–182.

Prentice, R. L. (1974). A log gamma model and its maximum likelihood estimation. *Biometrika 61*(3), 539–544.

Prentice, R. L. and L. A. Gloeckler (1978). Regression analysis of grouped survival data with application to breast cancer data. *Biometrics*, 57–67.

Rathore, A. S. and R. Mhatre (2011). *Quality by Design for Biopharmaceuticals: Principles and Case Studies*, Volume 1. John Wiley & Sons.

Ray, C. A., V. Patel, J. Shih, C. Macaraeg, Y. Wu, T. Thway, M. Ma, J. W. Lee, and B. DeSilva (2009). Application of multi-factorial design of experiments to successfully optimize immunoassays for robust measurements of therapeutic proteins. *Journal of Pharmaceutical and Biomedical Analysis 49*(2), 311–318.

Riegelman, R. and R. Hirsch (1989). *Studying a Study and Testing a Test: How to Read the Medical Literature*. Little Brown.

Ritz, C. (2010). Toward a unified approach to dose–response modeling in ecotoxicology. *Environmental Toxicology and Chemistry 29*(1), 220–229.

Rondeau, V., D. Commenges, and P. Joly (2003). Maximum penalized likelihood estimation in a gamma-frailty model. *Lifetime Data Analysis 9*(2), 139–153.

Rondeau, V., Y. Mazroui, and J. R. Gonzalez (2012). `frailtypack`: an R package for the analysis of correlated survival data with frailty models using penalized likelihood estimation or parametrical estimation. *Journal of Statistical Software 47*(4), 1–28.

Rosenberg, A. S. and A. Worobec (2004a). A risk-based approach to immunogenicity concerns of therapeutic protein products, part 1. *Biopharm International 17*(11), 22–26.

Rosenberg, A. S. and A. Worobec (2004b). A risk-based approach to immunogenicity concerns of therapeutic protein products, part 2: Considering host-specific and product-specific factors impacting immunogenicity. *Biopharm International 17*(12), 34–42.

Rosenberg, A. S. and A. Worobec (2005). A risk-based approach to immunogenicity concerns of therapeutic protein products, part 3: Effects of manufacturing changes in immunogenicity and the utility of animal immunogenicity studies. *Biopharm International*.

Rubbert-Roth, A. (2012). Assessing the safety of biologic agents in patients with rheumatoid arthritis. *Rheumatology 51*(suppl 5), v38–v47.

Sahu, S. K., D. K. Dey, and M. D. Branco (2003). A new class of multivariate skew distributions with applications to Bayesian regression models. *Canadian Journal of Statistics 31*(2), 129–150.

Satterthwaite, F. E. (1946). An approximate distribution of estimates of variance components. *Biometrics Bulletin*, 110–114.

Schlain, B., L. Amaravadi, J. Donley, A. Wickramasekera, D. Bennett, and M. Subramanyam (2010). A novel gamma-fitting statistical method for anti-drug antibody assays to establish assay cut points for data with non-normal distribution. *Journal of Immunological Methods 352*(1-2), 161–168.

Schuirmann, D. J. (1987). A comparison of the two one-sided tests procedure and the power approach for assessing the equivalence of average bioavailability. *Journal of Pharmacokinetics and Biopharmaceutics 15*(6), 657–680.

Shankar, G., S. Arkin, L. Cocea, V. Devanarayan, S. Kirshner, A. Krominga, V. Quarmby, S. Richards, C. Schneider, M. Subramanyam, et al. (2014). Assessment and reporting of the clinical immunogenicity of therapeutic proteins and peptides–harmonized terminology and tactical recommendations. *The AAPS Journal*, 1–16.

Shankar, G., V. Devanarayan, L. Amaravadi, Y. C. Barrett, R. Bowsher, D. Finco-Kent, M. Fiscella, B. Gorovits, S. Kirschner, and M. Moxness (2008). Recommendations for the validation of immunoassays used for detection of host antibodies against biotechnology products. *Journal of Pharmaceutical and Biomedical Analysis 48*(5), 1267–1281.

Shankar, G., C. Pendley, and K. E. Stein (2007). A risk-based bioanalytical strategy for the assessment of antibody immune responses against biological drugs. *Nature Biotechnology 25*(5), 555–561.

Shapiro, S. S. and M. B. Wilk (1965). An analysis of variance test for normality (complete samples). *Biometrika*, 591–611.

Shen, M., X. Dong, and Y. Tsong (2015). Statistical evaluation of several methods for cut point determination of immunogenicity screening assay. *Journal of Biopharmaceutical Statistics 25*(2), 269–279.

Shu, Y. (1997). *A SAS Macro for the Positive Stable Frailty Model*. Medical College of Wisconsin.

Snedecor, G. and W. Cochran (1989). *Statistical Methods*. Iowa State University Press, USA.

So, Y., G. Johnston, and S.-H. Him (2010). Analyzing interval-censored survival data with SAS software. SAS Global Forum.

Southworth, H. (2008). Statistically guided review of safety data in clinical trials. *PhUSE* (ST09).

Spiegelhalter, D. J., N. G. Best, B. P. Carlin, and A. Van Der Linde (2002). Bayesian measures of model complexity and fit. *Journal of the Royal Statistical Society: Series B (Statistical Methodology) 64*(4), 583–639.

Stangl, D. and D. Berry (2000). *Meta-Analysis in Medicine and Health Policy*. Chapman & Hall/CRC Biostatistics Series. Taylor & Francis.

Stollar, B. D. and E. W. Voss (1986). Antibodies to DNA. *Critical Reviews in Biochemistry and Molecular Biology 20*(1), 1–36.

Su, J., P. Sun, X. Li, and A. H. Hartford (2009). Fitting compartmental models to multiple dose pharmacokinetic data using SAS® PROC NLMIXED.

Subramanyam, M. (2008). Case study: immunogenicity of Natalizumab. In M. d. Weert and E. H. Møller (Eds.), *Immunogenicity of Biopharmaceuticals*, pp. 173–187. Springer.

Sun, J. (1995a). Empirical estimation of a distribution function with truncated and doubly interval-censored data and its application to aids studies. *Biometrics 51*(3), 1096–1104.

Sun, J. (1995b). Empirical estimation of a distribution function with truncated and doubly interval-censored data and its application to aids studies. *Biometrics*, 1096–1104.

Sun, J. (1996). A non-parametric test for interval-censored failure time data with application to AIDS studies. *Statistics in Medicine 15*(13), 1387–1395.

Sun, J. (1998). Interval censoring. *Encyclopedia of Biostatistics*, 2090–2095.

Sun, J. (2001). Nonparametric test for doubly interval-censored failure time data. *Lifetime Data Analysis 7*(4), 363–375.

Sun, J., Q. Liao, and M. Pagano (1999). Regression analysis of doubly censored failure time data with applications to aids studies. *Biometrics 55*(3), 909–914.

Tatarewicz, S., M. Moxness, D. Weeraratne, L. Zhou, M. Hale, S. J. Swanson, and N. Chirmule (2009). A step-wise approach for transfer of immunogenicity assays during clinical drug development. *The AAPS Journal 11*(3), 526–534.

Thornton, A. and P. Lee (2000). Publication bias in meta-analysis: its causes and consequences. *Journal of Clinical Epidemiology 53*(2), 207–216.

Turnbull, B. W. (1976). The empirical distribution function with arbitrarily grouped, censored and truncated data. *Journal of the Royal Statistical Society, Series B 38*, 290–295.

USP. Chapter<1106>: Immunogenicity assays– design and validation of immunoassays to detect anti-drug antibodies. *United States Pharmacopeia*.

van de Weert, M. and E. H. Møller (2008). *Immunogenicity of Biopharmaceuticals*, Volume 8. Springer.

Vander Heyden, Y., A. Nijhuis, J. Smeyers-Verbeke, B. Vandeginste, and D. Massart (2001). Guidance for robustness/ruggedness tests in method validation. *Journal of Pharmaceutical and Biomedical Analysis 24*(5), 723–753.

Vandermeer, B., L. Bialy, N. Hooton, L. Hartling, T. P. Klassen, B. C. Johnston, and N. Wiebe (2009, Aug). Meta-analyses of safety data: A comparison of exact versus asymptotic methods. *Statistical Methods in Medical Research 18*(4), 421–432.

Viechtbauer, W. (2010). Conducting meta-analyses in R with the `metafor` package. *Journal of Statistical Software 36*(3), 1–48.

Wadhwa, M., C. Bird, P. Dilger, R. Gaines-Das, and R. Thorpe (2003). Strategies for detection, measurement and characterization of unwanted antibodies induced by therapeutic biologicals. *Journal of Immunological Methods 278*(1), 1–17.

Wakshull, E. and D. Coleman (2011). Confirmatory immunogenicity assays. In M. G. Tovey (Ed.), *Detection and Quantification of Antibodies to Biopharmaceuticals: Practical and Applied Considerations*, pp. 103–117. Wiley.

Walker, E., A. V. Hernandez, and M. W. Kattan (2008). Meta-analysis: Its strengths and limitations. *Cleveland Clinic Journal of Medicine 75*(6), 431–439.

Wang, W., E. Zhi, and I. Chan (2002). Comparison of methods to analyze coarse immunogenicity data. In *ASA Proceedings of the Joint Statistical Meetings*, Alexandria, VA, pp. 3603–3608. American Statistical Association.

Wang, X., D. M. Morgan, G. Wang, and N. M. Mozier (2012). Residual DNA analysis in biologics development: Review of measurement and quantitation technologies and future directions. *Biotechnology and Bioengineering 109*(2), 307–317.

Wedderburn, R. W. (1974). Quasi-likelihood functions, generalized linear models, and the GaussNewton method. *Biometrika 61*(3), 439–447.

Wellner, J. A. and Y. Zhan (1997). A hybrid algorithm for computation of the nonparametric maximum likelihood estimator from censored data. *Journal of the American Statistical Association 92*(439), 945–959.

Westfall, P. H., D. V. Zaykin, and S. S. Young (2002). Multiple tests for genetic effects in association studies. In *Biostatistical Methods*, pp. 143–168. Springer.

Whitehead, A. (2002). *Meta-Analysis of Controlled Clinical Trials*. John Wiley & Sons.

Whitten, B. and A. Cohen (1986). Modified moment estimation for the three-parameter gamma distribution. *J. Qual. Technol.;(United States) 18*.

Wolbink, G. J., L. A. Aarden, and B. Dijkmans (2009). Dealing with immunogenicity of biologicals: assessment and clinical relevance. *Current Opinion in Rheumatology 21*(3), 211–215.

Wood, S. (2006). *Generalized Additive Models: An Introduction with R*. Chapman & Hall/CRC Texts in Statistical Science. Taylor & Francis.

Xia, H., H. Ma, and B. P. Carlin (2011). Bayesian hierarchical modeling for detecting safety signals in clinical trials. *Journal of Biopharmaceutical Statistics 21*(5), 1006–1029.

Yang, H. (2013). Setting specifications of correlated quality attributes through multivariate statistical modelling. *PDA Journal of Pharmaceutical Science and Technology 67*(5), 533–543.

Yang, H., Z. Wei, and M. Schenerman (2015). A statistical approach to determining criticality of residual host cell DNA. *Journal of Biopharmaceutical Statistics 25*(2), 234–246.

Yang, H., L. Zhang, and M. Galinski (2010). A probabilistic model for risk assessment of residual host cell DNA in biological products. *Vaccine 28*(19), 3308–3311.

Yu, B. (2006). Estimation of shared gamma frailty models by a modified EM algorithm. *Computational Statistics and Data Analysis 50*(2), 463 – 474.

Yu, K. H., R. L. Nation, and M. J. Dooley (2005). Multiplicity of medication safety terms, definitions and functional meanings: When is enough enough? *Quality and Safety in Health Care 14*(5), 358–363.

Zaccaro, D. and L. Aertker (2011). Use of zero-inflated mixture models to compare antibody titers in response to H1N1 vaccination. *Biopharmaceutical Report 18*(2), 17–26.

Zeger, S. L. and K.-Y. Liang (1986). Longitudinal data analysis for discrete and continuous outcomes. *Biometrics*, 121–130.

Zeger, S. L., K.-Y. Liang, and P. S. Albert (1988). Models for longitudinal data: a generalized estimating equation approach. *Biometrics*, 1049–1060.

Zelen, M. (1971). The analysis of several 2×2 contingency tables. *Biometrika 58*(1), 129–137.

Zhang, B. and S. Horvath (2005). A general framework for weighted gene co-expression network analysis. *Statistical Applications in Genetics and Molecular Biology 4*(1).

Zhang, J., B. Yu, L. Zhang, L. Roskos, L. Richman, and H. Yang (2015). Non-normal random effects models for immunogenicity assay cut point determination. *Journal of Biopharmaceutical Statistics 25*(2), 295–306.

Zhang, J., L. Zhang, and H. Yang (2014). Sample size consideration for immunoassay screening cut-point determination. *Journal of Biopharmaceutical Statistics 24*(3), 535–545.

Zhang, L., J. J. Zhang, R. J. Kubiak, and H. Yang (2013). Statistical methods and tool for cut point analysis in immunogenicity assays. *Journal of Immunological Methods 389*(1), 79–87.

Zhang, P., P. X.-K. Song, A. Qu, and T. Greene (2008). Efficient estimation for patient-specific rates of disease progression using nonnormal linear mixed models. *Biometrics 64*(1), 29–38.

Zhang, W., J. Liu, Y. Q. Niu, L. Wang, and X. Hu (2008). A Bayesian regression approach to the prediction of MHC-II binding affinity. *Computer Methods and Programs in Biomedicine 92*(1), 1–7.

Zhao, Q. and J. Sun (2004). Generalized log-rank test for mixed interval-censored failure time data. *Statistics in Medicine 23*(10), 1621–1629.

Zhong, J., K. Lee, and Y. Tsong (2008). Statistical assessment of analytical method transfer. *Journal of Biopharmaceutical Statistics 18*(5), 1005–1012.

Zhong, Z. D., S. Dinnogen, M. Hokom, C. Ray, D. Weinreich, S. J. Swanson, and N. Chirmule (2010). Identification and inhibition of drug target interference in immunogenicity assays. *Journal of Immunological Methods 355*(1), 21–28.

Zhong, Z. D. and L. Zhou (2013). Good practices for statistical estimation of cut point. In R. Dodge and R. Pillutla (Eds.), *Immunogenicity Assay Development, Validation and Implementation*. London: Future Science.

Zhou, M., L. Lee, and K. Chen (2003). Compute the NPMLE of distribution from doubly censored data. *Analysis*, 9.

Zink, R. C. (2013). Assessing drug safety with Bayesian hierarchical modeling usign PROC MCMC and JMP. *Pharmaceutical SAS Users Group* (179).

Index